TOUCH & STRETCH

TOUCH & STRETCH:
Shiatsu for Everyone

TORU NAMIKOSHI

Japan Publications, Inc.

Published by Japan Publications, Inc., Tokyo

Distributors:
UNITED STATES: Kodansha America, Inc., through Oxford University Press,
198 Madison Avenue, New York, N.Y. 10016. CANADA: Fitzhenry &
Whiteside Ltd., 195 Allstate Parkway, Markham, Ontario L3R 4T8. UNITED
KINGDOM AND EUROPEAN CONTINENT: Premier Book Marketing Ltd.,
1 Gower Street, London WC1E 6HA. AUSTRALIA AND NEW ZEALAND:
Bookwise International, 54 Crittenden Road, Findon, South Australia 5023.
ASIA AND JAPAN: Japan Publications Trading Co., Ltd., 1−2−1, Sarugaku-
cho, Chiyoda−ku, Tokyo 101-0064 Japan

First edition: April 1985
Seventh printing: April 2000

ISBN 4−8170−9004−9

Originally published in 1985 as "Shiatsu + Stretching "

Printed in U.S.A.

Preface

Ever since man stood on two legs and walked erect, unlike the quadrupeds, owing to the weight of head and torso, he has been fated to suffer from stiff shoulders and lumbago. To prevent or treat these conditions, human beings perform various movements to limber their bodies; and, from ancient times, different kinds of manual therapy have been combined with these motions in a wide variety of health and exercise regimens.

The combination of shiatsu with currently popular stretching arose from the same kind of need and has been systematized into the form set forth in this book. Neither shiatsu nor stretching requires much space. Both can be performed quietly and leisurely anytime and anywhere. The two are, therefore, perfectly suited to the needs of modern people, especially those who live in crowded cities and whose work requires them to be stationary in more or less the same posture for long periods.

Shiatsu and stretching evolve from perfectly instinctive actions executed to ease discomfort or relax the body. Without knowing it, the person who strokes, presses, or kneads a numb or sore muscle is performing shiatsu. And, the person who stretches arms and legs in bed in the morning or raises his arms above his head and bends his back after a long time in the same position is performing what today is called stretching.

The flexion and extension of back, arms, and legs with which we follow up shiatsu therapy fall into the stretching category. For instance, after performing shiatsu therapy on a patient who is lying prone, assuming a position facing the patient at his feet, I grip the ankle of the treated leg with both hands and, pulling toward myself, raise the leg from the floor and hold it in the raised and pulled position for ten seconds. In some instances, the stretched leg may be from one to four—or even five in extreme cases—centimeters longer than the other leg. Often stretching in this way has been known to relieve habitual cramping, sports-inflicted pain in the elbow, and abnormal spinal curvature.

And, from my experiences with such recovery, I came to think that shiatsu and stretching could be effectively combined. The desire to do so was the original motivation for this book.

Iwao Yoshizaki, president of Japan Publications, Inc, took an interest in the idea and encouraged me to begin writing. But labor pains were intense, and I deviated many times before I finally put my thoughts in well-organized form. I should like to express my deep gratitude to Mr. Yoshizaki and to Yotsuko Watanabe for patiently waiting for my manuscript and then for editing and ordering it after it was in their hands.

To employ a laundering metaphor, if shiatsu can be compared to washing clothes, stretching may be likened to the ironing that smooths out all wrinkles. I hope that this book will help many people understand that, combined, as they are presented here, the two can do a great deal to improve health and appearance, to increase the effectiveness of sports training, and to prevent aging.

TORU NAMIKOSHI

Contents

8

Chapter Three: Therapeutic Applications

Names of Parts and Zones of the Human Body (Anterior Surface)

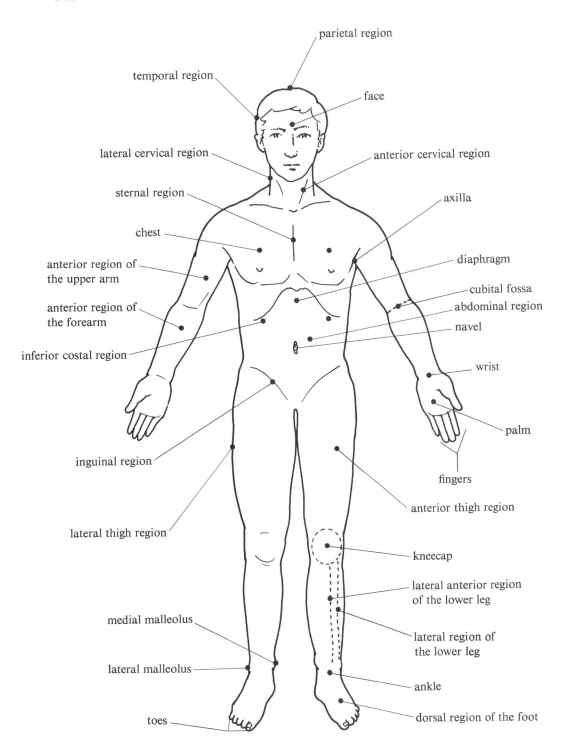

parietal region

temporal region

face

lateral cervical region

anterior cervical region

sternal region

axilla

chest

anterior region of the upper arm

diaphragm

cubital fossa

anterior region of the forearm

abdominal region

navel

inferior costal region

wrist

palm

inguinal region

fingers

anterior thigh region

lateral thigh region

kneecap

lateral anterior region of the lower leg

medial malleolus

lateral region of the lower leg

lateral malleolus

ankle

toes

dorsal region of the foot

Names of Parts and Zones of the Human Body (Posterior Surface)

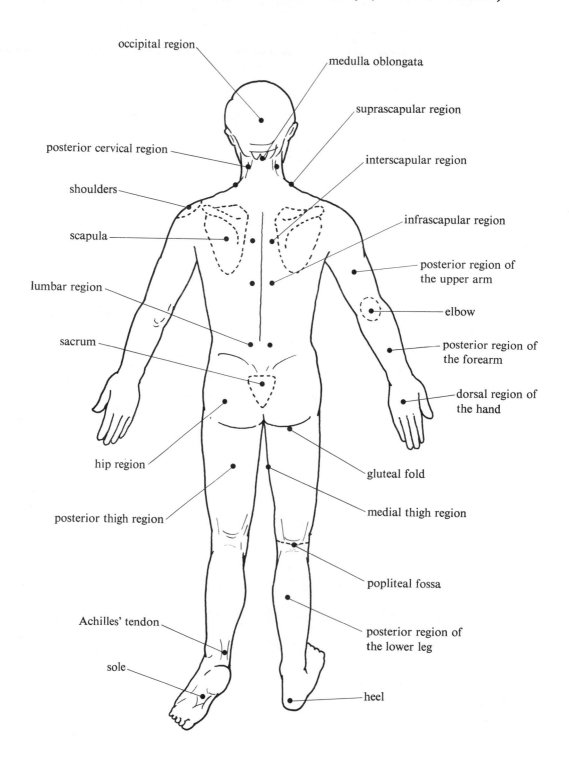

occipital region

medulla oblongata

suprascapular region

posterior cervical region

interscapular region

shoulders

scapula

infrascapular region

lumbar region

posterior region of the upper arm

elbow

sacrum

posterior region of the forearm

dorsal region of the hand

hip region

gluteal fold

posterior thigh region

medial thigh region

popliteal fossa

Achilles' tendon

posterior region of the lower leg

sole

heel

Chapter One

General Principles

1. Shiatsu and Stretching

The Significance of Shiatsu Therapy

Unconsciously, whenever they feel sluggishness, stiffness, numbness or pain in some part of the body, human beings stroke or press the affected area with the hands. Actions of this kind are instinctive attempts to cure disorders and predate medicine and history itself. Japanese words for treatment (*teatè*) and for conditions that have gotten completely out of hand (*te-okurè*) both include the word for hand (*te*) and suggest the ancient therapeutic importance of manual manipulation. Though they may differ in method, both Western massage and oriental *amma* massage derive from the instinctive use of the hands in curing.

Amma, which originated in China and passed into Japan, was long popular among the people because of its convenience. It reached a peak of popularity during the Edo period (1600–1867). With the influx of Western culture that followed the opening of Japan in the second half of the nineteenth century, however, *amma* was to a large extent replaced by Western massage.

Though they differ in origin, therapeutic principles, methods, and effects, both *amma* and massage share certain features. They both employ rubbing, pounding, kneading, and stroking techniques executed rhythmically and quickly. Both are dynamic.

In contrast to them, the distinctively Japanese therapeutic method called *shiatsu*, as founded by Tokujirō Namikoshi, is calm in nature. It employs the digital balls of the fingers and thumbs and the thenars of the hands, parts of the body that are comparatively fleshy and soft. And its basic principle is to apply pressure to the surface of the body in a gradual way so that it penetrates and limbers the muscles beneath. This kind of treatment does not unduly stimulate or fatigue the muscles. It improves therapeutic effects by evoking the body's own natural powers of recuperation.

The modern system of shiatsu, founded on these principles, determines the points on the surface of the body that are most effective in such treatment from the standpoint of contemporary anatomy and physiology and devises the most suitable manual techniques for various parts of the body.

■ *Shiatsu therapy, the aim of which is the prevention and treatment of illness, is a system for improving health by removing fatigue-causing elements and stimulating the body's natural powers of recuperation by means of digital and manual pressure applied to certain established points on the surface of the body.*

The Significance of Stretching

Stretching, which must be performed slowly and without strain, extends the muscles as much as possible to maximize their flexion. Though some people tend to consider stretching therapy a newly evolved treatment, like shiatsu itself, it too derives from such instinctive human behavior as stretching the limbs, yawning, rubbing or popping the eyes, and so on upon waking in the morning. All of these actions are unconsciously performed warm-up exercises for the muscles and the whole body.

The modern stretching training system involves mainly actions that extend the mobile powers of muscles and joints. Differing from athletic warming-up training, which makes use of quick rhythm and rebound, stretching training extends parts of the body slowly in synchronization with calm breathing. When full muscular extension has been reached, the stretched position is held for a specified length of time. Correctly performed, stretching is highly effective and puts no undue burden on the muscles. Since it is not fatiguing, it may be comfortably carried out by the physically weak and elderly.

Excessive stretching, however, must be avoided. No doubt many of my readers will understand why if they recall the times when too violent stretching has caused cramps in the calves or when sudden and wide yawning has brought on pain in the root of the tongue and the lower jaw.

■ *Stretching exercises slowly extend the muscles, which are held in the stretched position for a specified amount of time. They constitute a system of training that increases the extension limits of muscles and joints, cultivates muscular power and endurance, and keeps the muscles limber.*

Cumulative Effects of Shiatsu+ Stretching

Shiatsu removes muscular stiffness, improves flexibility, and eliminates fatigue. Stretching extends the muscles, improves circulation, increases resilience, and strengthens the muscles. The two performed together combine the good effects of both.

As a rule, stretching follows thorough shiatsu. In this sense, shiatsu may be compared to warming-up, and stretching to sports activities. Engaging in rough and demanding sports without sufficient warm-up is to invite accident and injury. Similarly, performing stretching exercises without taking into consideration muscular fatigue and stiffness entails the risk of increasing fatigue and causing physical damage. Preceding stretching with thorough shiatsu, which limbers the muscles and eliminates fatigue, increases the range of extension and strengthens the muscles. When the muscles are pliant and strong, the range and smoothness of the mobility of the joints too will improve.

In this way, combining them complements and reinforces the effectiveness of both shiatsu and stretching. Furthermore, since neither of them takes much space, time, or physical strength, they can be performed at the individual's convenience. Making use of extra minutes in bath or bed or whatever leisure presents itself to carry out a program of shiatsu and stretching can relieve fatigue, strengthen the body, and make it possible to stay youthful and healthy longer.

2. Physical Effects of Shiatsu and Stretching

The Skin

The human skin alters with the passing of time from the rosy smoothness of infancy, to the vigorous tautness of adolescence, to the small wrinkles of middle age, to the deep creases of old age. The first step in staying youthful in appearance is to prevent aging of the skin.

The sweat glands and the sebaceous glands supply moisture and nutrition to the skin. The sweat glands ensure constant evaporation of water from the skin surface and at the same time rid the body of such wastes as carbon dioxide gas and fatigue-causing elements in the process known as dermal respiratiou. Death from such things as completely encasing the skin in some substance or in loss of as much of one-third of the skin as a consequence of burns occurs because of the body's loss of ability to eliminate wastes through this dermal process.

Located above the hair roots, the sebaceous glands secrete an oily substance supplied by the subcutaneous fat. Wrinkling and sagging of the skin in old age occur because the subcutaneous fat shrinks, thus hindering the secretion of oil by the sebaceous glands.

Shiatsu stimulates circulation in the capillaries of skin tissue, activates dermal cells, and invigorates secretion from the sebaceous glands. This in turn keeps the skin moist, smooth, and taut. At the same time it invigorates the skin surface, stimulating the secretion of the sweat glands and the elimination of wastes through them.

Stretching gives the skin resilience and helps prevent wrinkling. By activating its functioning, shiatsu and stretching together heighten the sensitivity of the skin and thus improve its ability to adjust body temperature to external temperature and prevent chills and colds.

Muscular System

Muscles in the human body are of the voluntary kind, which may be consciously controlled, and the involuntary kind, which may not. The skeletal muscles, which connect bones and control the posture and motion of the body and are composed of long, slender muscular fibers, are voluntary.

By contracting, they draw the two bones to which they are connected closer to each other. Though they play roles in various kinds of movements, their major ones are to bend and unbend joints. Flexor muscles bend joints and extensor one unbend, or extend, them. Both kinds work in mutual antagonism and are therefore called antagonist muscles. When one moves in one direction, the other moves in another. If they did not, it would be impossible to extend a joint once it had been bent. Antagonistic muscles are not limited to the flexors and extensors: among the several others are the supinator muscles that turn the wrist outward and the pronator muscles that turn it inward. Even when no motion is involved, the flexors and extensors work together to preserve bodily balance and to assist in maintaining posture or lifting things. Since all the muscles of the body are tensed even when the posture is one of inactivity and relax only during slumber, getting adequate sleep is obviously very important to preventing muscular fatigue.

Excess muscular tension and fatigue cause the muscle fibers to stiffen. This in turn reduces nourishment to an insufficient level by stagnating the circulation of blood and lymph. On the other hand, insufficient exercise weakens the metabolism thus reducing nourishment to the muscle tissues, causing the muscle fibers to become thin, and depriving the muscles of tone and power.

Shiatsu pressure applied from the surface penetrates the muscles, limbers them, and improves their nutrition by stimulating circulation of blood and lymph. By extending the muscle fibers, stretching makes contraction and extension smoother. Performed together, shiatsu and stretching thicken the muscle fibers, increase their powers of contraction, facilitate the movement of joints, and amplify muscular power and endurance.

Skeletal System

Calcium and other nutrients reach the backbone and all the other bones of the body by means of small holes, called nutrient foramens, at certain fixed locations. This and the proper supply of fluids to the bones are essential to good health. For instance, the intervertebral discs, which are eighty percent water, degenerate and deform if their supply of fluid and nutrients is insufficient.

To prevent such degeneration, the most important thing is to stimulate circulation and the flow of nutrients and thus to strengthen the bones. Shiatsu and stretching, especially on the back, produce this effect by limbering the muscles and thereby prevent pathological spinal curvature and degeneration of the intervertebral discs. Furthermore they facilitate the motion of the arm and leg joints and prevent deformation, arthritis, and pain in the joints.

Nervous System

Spread over the entire body and connecting all the internal organs is the nervous system, which may be divided into the central and the peripheral nervous systems. The central system, which consists of the cerebrum and the spinal cord, is the main trunk. The peripheral system is further subdivided into the cerebrospinal and the autonomic systems. Included in the cerebrospinal system are the motor nerves, which govern all motion, and the sensory nerves, which account for awareness to pain, heat, and cold.

The nerves transmit to the brain information about muscular fatigue. But, if they grow dull, such information is not forthcoming; and an irregularity in the muscles can be overlooked till it develops into a subjective symptom. Cramps, sprains, pulled muscles, and torn Achilles' tendons experienced by sportsmen are not sudden occurrences but the results of gradual hardening of the muscles and dulling of the nerves.

Frequent, regular shiatsu and stretching limber the muscles, prevent the accumulation of fatigue, and keep the nerves alert. By stimulating the motor nerves, they expedite transmission of information to the brain, act on the skeletal muscles, and increase the mobility range of the joints.

Circulatory System

If, in work or other activities, the same posture or position is maintained for a long time, circulation in some part of the body will be obstructed; and the muscles of the affected region will fail to get the nutrients they require. Under such circumstances, the feet, which are distant from the heart, swell. Practically everyone has noticed at one time or other that shoes seem tighter in the evening than they were in the morning of the same day. This is because the feet have swollen. Circulation is improved by immediate shiatsu and stretching to any part of the body where the muscles seem to have stiffened. It is especially important for people whose legs have weakened because of inactivity resulting from constant desk work to perform shiatsu and stretching daily to strengthen their limbs.

Alimentary System

By regulating the functioning of the digestive system, shiatsu on the abdominal region improves assimilation of food and in this way sustains nutritional balance and increases stamina by making possible effective storing of energy in the body. Stretching in the same region removes subcutaneous fat and limbers and strengthens the abdominal muscle group. In addition, it limbers the smooth (involuntary) muscles of the internal organs, thus improving functioning and preventing such abnormal lowering of the organs as gastroptosis.

Of course, in addition to shiatsu and stretching, it is of the utmost importance to maintain a balanced diet and to chew foods thoroughly. Chewing stimulates the secretion of saliva and thus facilitates digestion. Saliva contains a hormone called parotin, which retards the aging process.

Endocrine System

By secreting hormones directly into the bloodstream, by means of which they are carried to all organs, the endocrine system preserves the body's chemical balance. Reduced functioning of this system destroys hormone balance and causes various serious pathological conditions.

The medulla oblongata, located in the nuchal fossa between the occipital bone and the first cervical vertebra, is of the greatest importance in connection with shiatsu for the entire body. Shiatsu and stretching in this region affect the pituitary gland and help maintain bodily hormone balance.

Shiatsu on the right and left lateral cervical zones intensifies the functioning of the thyroid gland, which, located in front of the trachea, secretes hormones controlling metabolism.

The salivary hormone, contained in saliva, is related to the metabolism of bone tissues and the strengthening of bones. Saliva is secreted by the parotid, submaxillary, and sublingual glands. The secretions of these same glands affect the sex hormones, which control the reproductive system. Shiatsu and stretching centering on the mouth and jaws influence these glands.

Insulin, which plays the important role of reducing blood sugar, is secreted by the pancreas, deficient functioning of which is a major cause of diabetes. Shiatsu and stretching for the right and left infrascapular regions affect the pancreas and stimulate insulin secretion.

The suprarenal glands, located above the right and left kidneys, consist of cortex and medullary substance. The medullary substance, which affects the sympathetic nervous system, stimulates contraction of the blood vessels and secretes adrenaline which responds to stress. The cortex secretes several tens of different hormones, all of which are important to the body's immunity system. The kidneys themselves preserve balance in the blood by removing wastes from the body in the form of urine. Shiatsu and stretching on the infrascapular and lumbar regions stimulate the functioning of the suprarenal glands and kidneys, thus improving resistance, increasing muscular strength, and maintaining balance among the components of the blood.

Sex hormones secreted by the testes and the ovaries regulate the reproductive functions and account for the characteristic masculine and feminine traits of the sexes. Shiatsu and stretching on the lower abdomen, the sacral region, and the Namikoshi points (see p. 62) affect these glands and regulate the reproductive system.

Five Rules for Shiatsu and Stretching

1. Relax the body. Perform stretching only after thorough shiatsu has limbered the muscles.
2. Both shiatsu and stretching must be performed gradually and in synchronization with the breathing. No violent or excessively lively action is called for.
3. Heighten the effectiveness of treatment by adjusting the strength of shiatsu pressure and the length of time stretching postures are held to the condition of the muscles being treated. To this end, an accurate

understanding of such conditions is essential.

4. Always urinate and defecate before initiating treatment.

5. Make daily treatment more fun by drawing up a varied program combining shiatsu and stretching according to your own needs and goals.

When Not to Perform Shiatsu and Stretching

1. On an empty stomach or immediately after eating.

2. When you have a fever.

3. When you have an external injury to the skin, concussion, sprain, or an incompletely knit broken bone.

4. When in poor or extremely weak condition.

5. Immediately after suffering the whiplash syndrome in a traffic accident.

6. When suffering inflammation in an internal organ or ulcers.

7. When drinking alcohol or smoking.

17

3. Shiatsu Techniques

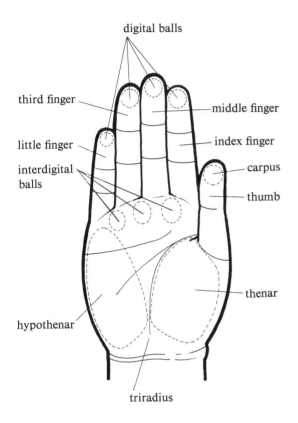

Use of Hands and Fingers

● *One Thumb*
The digital ball of one thumb is pressed against the skin, and the other four fingers are held together and placed lightly on the body as support (Fig. 1). For use in treating the left and right anterior cervical region, the back, the Namikoshi points, the arms, the palms, the legs, and the soles of the feet.

Fig. 1 One-thumb Pressure

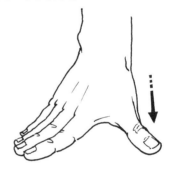

● *Both Thumbs*
The outer sides of the tips of both thumbs are held together, and the digital balls are pressed against the skin. The other four fingers of each hand provide light support. Pressure is applied with both thumbs simultaneously (Fig. 2). For use in treating the back, the legs, and the soles of the feet.

Fig. 2 Two-thumb Pressure

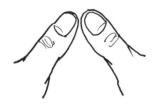

● *Overlapped Thumbs*
In general, the right thumb is on the bottom; and the left one is on top, pressed against its fingernail. The other four fingers of each hand are used for light support. Pressure is applied with both thumbs simultaneously (Fig. 3). This is used when strong pressure is desirable. For use in treating the back, the legs, and the soles of the feet.

Fig. 3 Overlapped-thumb Pressure

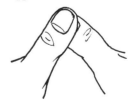

● *Index, Middle, and Fourth Fingers*
The thumbs serve as support, and the digital balls of the index, middle, and fourth fingers are pressed against the skin (Fig. 4). For use in treating the head, the face, the lateral cervical region, the posterior cervical region, the supra-scapular region, the chest, and the abdomen.

Fig. 4   Single-finger Pressure

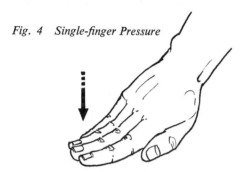

● *Overlapped Palms*
With both hands turned in the same direction, the palm of one is pressed against the skin; and the palm of the other is placed on top of the lower hand. When a person is giving himself shiatsu pressure, the hands should be turned in opposite directions. Pressure is applied as it is with one palm only (Fig. 6). For use in treating the head and the abdomen.

Fig. 7   Interlocked-hand Pressure

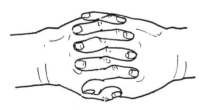

● *Opposed Thumb and Fingers*
The digital ball of the thumb is held opposite the digital balls of the other four fingers. The part of the patient's body being treated is gripped between thumb and fingers (Fig. 8). For use in treating the arms, legs, calves, and Achilles' tendons.

● *Palm*
The fingers and the entire palm of the hand are pressed against the skin (Fig. 5). For use in treating the head, the eyes, the shoulder joints, the back, and the knees.

Fig. 5   One-palm Pressure

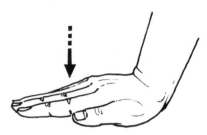

Fig. 6   Overlapped-palm Pressure

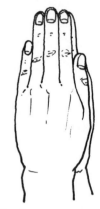

● *Interlocked Hands*
The fingers of the hands are interlocked, and the carpal regions of both are pressed against the skin. Pressure is applied with both hands simultaneously (Fig. 7). For use in treating the head, the back, and the right and left kidney regions.

Fig. 8   Pressure with Opposed Thumb and Four Fingers

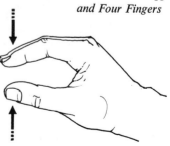

*Fig. 9 Pressure with Opposed Thumb and Index
Finger*

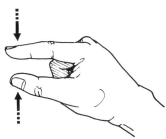

• *Thenar (Radial Carpal Ball)*
The thenar of the hand is pressed against the
skin (Fig. 10). For use in treating the face and
the inguinal region.

• *Overlapped Index and Middle Fingers*
For stability, the tip of the middle finger is
pressed on top of the fingernail of the index
finger. The other fingers are held lightly closed.
Pressure is applied with the tip of the index
finger on the bottom (Fig. 11). For use in treating the sides of the nose and the face.

Fig. 12 Pressure with Overlapped Middle Fingers

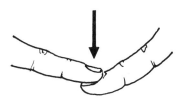

• *Opposed Thumb and Index Finger*
Similar to the preceding except that the part of
the patient's body being treated is gripped
between the digital balls of the thumb and the
index finger (Fig. 9). For use in treating the
fingers, toes, and Achilles' tendons.

Fig. 10 Thenar Pressure

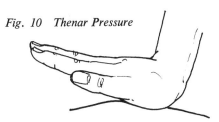

*Fig. 11 Pressure with Overlapped Index and Middle
Fingers*

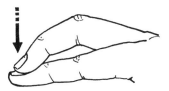

• *Overlapped Middle Fingers*
All fingers except the middle fingers of both
hands are lightly closed. The tip of one middle
finger is placed on the fingernail of the other.
Pressure is applied with the digital balls of both
fingers (Fig. 12). For use in treating the medulla
oblongata.

Types of Pressure Application

Fig. 13 Standard Pressure

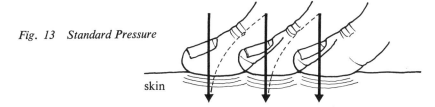

skin

• *Standard*
In this most frequently employed method,
steady pressure is applied perpendicular to the
surface of the body (Fig. 13). Each application

lasts from three to five seconds. Pressure is
gently released before the next application is
initiated. Before applying pressure, inhale.
Then exhale as you press.

• *Graded Pressure*

Pressure is applied in three grades—light, medium, and strong—and a stop is made between the second and third stages (Fig. 14). First move from light to medium pressure and hold that for the specified amount of time. Then, without removing the fingertips from the surface of the skin, release pressure. Finally, move on to strong pressure. Each application should last from three to seven seconds. In some instances, application durations too are graded; three, five, and seven seconds.

Fig. 14   Graded Pressure

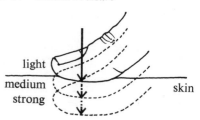

• *Sustained Pressure*

Generally applied with the palm or palms, after reaching a certain level of intensity, this kind of pressure is maintained for from five to ten seconds (Fig. 15).

Fig. 15   Sustained Pressure

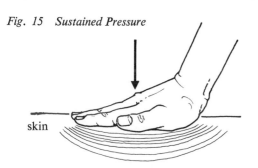

Maintain steady pressure

• *Concentrated Pressure*

Pressure is applied, usually with overlapped thumbs, to one shiatsu point for from five to seven seconds with gradually increasing intensity until a certain level is reached. Then, with the finger still against the skin, the pressure is gradually released and then applied once again (Fig. 16). This is repeated several times.

Fig. 16   Concentrated Pressure

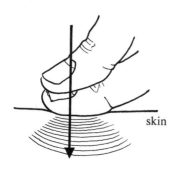

• *Suction Pressure*

In this special technique, the fingers (or palm), placed close against the skin, are used to pull, in a sucking fashion and usually toward the person performing shiatsu, the connective tissues between skin and muscles (Fig. 17).

• *Flowing Pressure*

Employing either the palm or the fingers, this kind of pressure application moves rhythmically and in a flowing fashion forward and backward or right and left from point to point (Fig. 18). Pressure on each point lasts for from one to two seconds.

Fig. 17   Suction Pressure

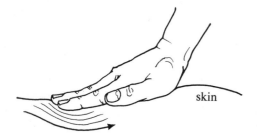

Fig. 18   Flowing Pressure

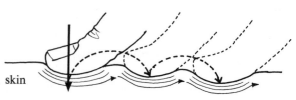

• *Vibration*

Small-frequency vibrations and very low pressure are applied to the patient's body by lightly placing fingers (or palm) against the skin and moving them back and forth (Fig. 19). The characteristics of this technique are the pleasant

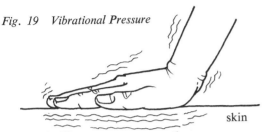

Fig. 19   Vibrational Pressure

skin

sensation it produces and the depth to which its effects penetrate.

• *Palm Stimulus*

In this technique, as steady pressure is maintained, the palm, which is pressed tight against the skin, strokes the body downward quickly (Fig. 20). It is used mainly on the abdomen or the spinal column to stimulate the spinal nerves. The technique may be executed with one palm only, with overlapped palms, or with one palm placed on top of and at right angles to the other hand.

Fig. 20   Palm-stimulation Pressure

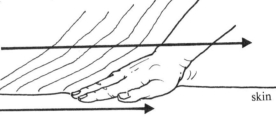

skin

Intensity Control

To regulate shiatsu-pressure intensity it is essential to have an accurate understanding of the condition of the muscles under treatment. Gauging pressure by muscle stiffness will increase the effectiveness of therapy and make a steady difference in the way in which the muscles can be limbered.

Applying sudden, strong pressure to very stiff muscles has only adverse effects. If, on the other hand, gentle pressure, interspersed with occasional applications of strong pressure, is used, treatment will be effective.

As time passes, the person performing shiatsu will come to understand the changes taking place in muscular condition. When this happens, he should vary pressures and suit the application techniques and the parts of the hands used to the needs of the moment.

• *Stages of Pressure Intensity*

Touch.   Bare contact between the skin and the hands. Touching, which should last three seconds for each point, may be used in tactile diagnoses to determine whether a part of the body is feverish or chilled.

Slight Pressure.   The patient should have a soft sense of pressure on the skin. Application lasts three seconds for each point. Applied to connective tissues between skin and muscle, this kind of pressure is used to detect roughness, moisture, and stiffness and to determine skin tone.

Light Pressure.   A little stronger than the preceding, this kind of pressure lasts three to five seconds for each point. It penetrates very lightly through the skin and to the surfaces of the muscles. In this way, it helps determine muscular resilience and pliancy.

Medium Pressure.   Slightly stronger than the preceding, this kind of pressure, which is applied from three to six seconds for each point, detects muscular stiffness. It is pleasant because its effects reach deep into the muscles.

Strong Pressure. The strongest employed in shiatsu, this kind of pressure extends deep to the central parts of stiff muscles. It may be pleasingly painful, but must be no stronger than can be easily endured. It lasts three to seven seconds for each point.

4. Stretching Techniques

Before stretching is begun, it is essential to attain mental unity by breathing deeply and regulating the breath. This will relax the muscles and prepare the body for the positions in which stretching is to be performed.

● *Durations*
Though muscular condition influences it, in general the duration of each stretched position ranges from ten seconds to a maximum of thirty seconds. In all cases, it is essential to understand muscular condition and gauge stretching duration to it. Even when instructions in this book call for fifteen seconds, if the muscles are very stiff and holding the position as long as that is difficult, the period may be shortened to twelve or thirteen or even ten seconds. Gradually, as stretching is continued, the muscles will limber, making longer durations possible.

● *Postures*
The postures explained in the text must be thoroughly understood and accurately executed. The body must be in a correctly balanced posture for stretching exercises. Forcing the body into poorly balanced positions for a long period of time can cause disorders. None of the stretching positions in which the head is held low should be maintained for longer than ten seconds at a time.

● *Alternating Shiatsu and Stretching*
Always limber the muscles thoroughly by shiatsu treatment before undertaking stretching exercises. And use further shiatsu to limber muscles that have tensed and stiffened owing to repeated stretching. Stretching may then be continued. Alternating shiatsu and stretching in this way prevents undue stress on muscles.

● *Simultaneous Shiatsu and Stretching*
In some parts of the body it is possible to stretch while performing shiatsu and perform shiatsu while stretching. For instance, it is permissible to carry out dorsiflexion and plantarflexion stretching of the toes and soles while performing shiatsu on the lower legs. Or, since both hands remain idle while the lower legs are being stretched, it is possible to perform shiatsu on the back or lumbar region at the same time. Each person may work out the combinations of the two that are most effective for his individual needs and goals.

1. Warming-up

Traditionally, rubbing the hands together symbolizes the merchant who is eager to sell something to a customer. Medically, however, this same rubbing of the hands concentrates and improves circulation in the fingers and calms the brain. Improving circulation limbers the fingers and intensifies the tactile sensitivity of the fingertips. This in turn enables the person performing shiatsu to judge accurately the conditions of the patient's skin and muscles and gauge the degree of pressure being applied. Consequently, executing these warm-up exercises for the hands and fingers before initiating it greatly enhances the effectiveness of shiatsu or stretching therapy.

As shall be discussed later, there are reflex points on the fingers and palms that relate to the internal organs. Shiatsu and stretching performed with the fingers and palms stimulate reflexes that invigorate the functioning of those organs.

Though, in the following explanations of warm-up exercises, sometimes instructions are given for one hand only, it is always necessary to carry out the same procedures on the other hand as well.

• *Wrists*
Warming-up for the joints begins with limbering the wrists. Three rows of six shiatsu points each

lie from the middle of the forearm to the wrist on the palmar side of the arm. One row is in line with the little finger, one with the middle finger, and one with the thumb. Press each for three seconds. Repeat three times (Figs. 1 and 2). After thorough shiatsu, bend the wrist inward (palmar flexion) ninety degrees and hold this stretched position ten seconds; repeat three times (Fig. 3).

Fig. 1

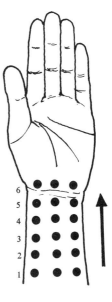

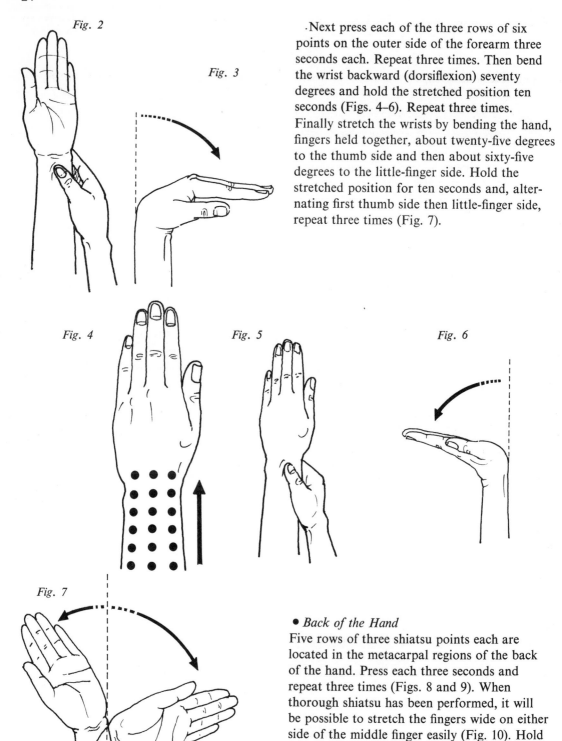

Fig. 2

Fig. 3

Fig. 4

Fig. 5

Fig. 6

Fig. 7

·Next press each of the three rows of six points on the outer side of the forearm three seconds each. Repeat three times. Then bend the wrist backward (dorsiflexion) seventy degrees and hold the stretched position ten seconds (Figs. 4–6). Repeat three times. Finally stretch the wrists by bending the hand, fingers held together, about twenty-five degrees to the thumb side and then about sixty-five degrees to the little-finger side. Hold the stretched position for ten seconds and, alternating first thumb side then little-finger side, repeat three times (Fig. 7).

● *Back of the Hand*
Five rows of three shiatsu points each are located in the metacarpal regions of the back of the hand. Press each three seconds and repeat three times (Figs. 8 and 9). When thorough shiatsu has been performed, it will be possible to stretch the fingers wide on either side of the middle finger easily (Fig. 10). Hold this stretched position ten seconds and repeat three times.

Fig. 8

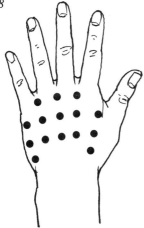

Fig. 9

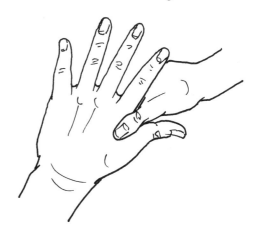

Fig. 10

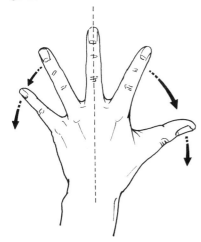

● *Palm of the Hand*
Four rows of three shiatsu points each lie on the palm of the hand in the metacarpal regions from the wrist to the bases of the fingers (Fig. 11). Press each point for three seconds. Repeat three times. When thorough shiatsu had been completed, close the fingers, pressing those on either side firmly against the middle finger (Fig. 12). There must be no gaps between fingers. Hold this position ten seconds and repeat three times.

Fig. 11

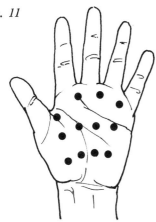

Fig. 12

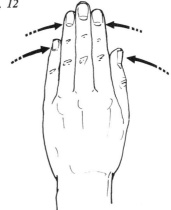

Fig. 13

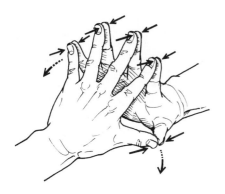

Fig. 14

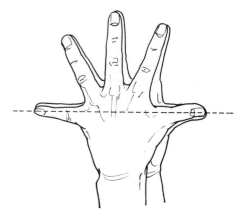

• *Two-hand Stretching for the Metacarpal Regions*

Place the digital balls of thumb, index, middle, fourth, and little fingers of one hand against the digital balls of the corresponding fingers of the other hand and, pressing them against each other, gradually spread the fingers till the

thumbs and little fingers form a straight, horizontal line (Figs. 13 and 14). It is important that contact be made only between digital balls. Hold this stretched position for ten seconds and repeat three times.

• *Two-hand Stretching for the Wrists*

Pressing the fingers and palm of one hand against the fingers and palm of the other, extend the arms straight forward. Stretch by turning both hands first in the direction of the thumb (radial deviation) and then in the direction of the little finger (ulnar deviation; Figs. 15 and 16). Hold each stretched position ten seconds and repeat three times.

Next, in the same position, bend both wrists first to the right and then to the left (Fig. 17). Hold each stretched position ten seconds and repeat three times. This exercise involves plantar flexion and dorsiflexion for each wrist in alternation.

Fig. 15

Fig. 16

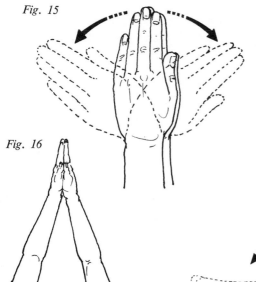

Fig. 17

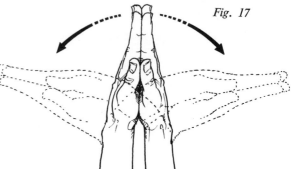

Fig. 18

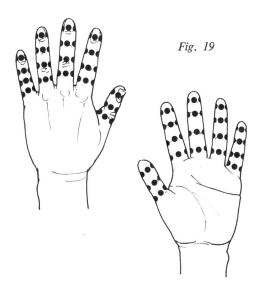

Fig. 19

Fig. 20

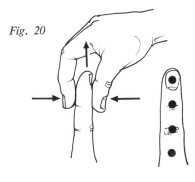

Fig. 21

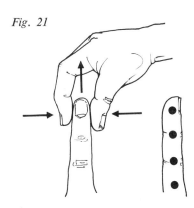

● *Fingers*

Holding each finger from the front and back between thumb and index finger execute shiatsu on the three points on the thumb and the four points on all the other fingers (Figs. 18 and 19). Work from the lowest points to those at the tips of the fingers. Press each point for three seconds. On each finger, pressure on the final point at the tip should be accompanied by an upward pull (Fig. 20). No repetition is necessary.

After pressing each point from front and back, press again on the same locations from both sides of each finger. Press all points once for three seconds each, giving the final points an upward pull (Fig. 21). No repetition is necessary.

● *Finger-alignment Stretching*

Standing with the elbows slightly bent and the fingers of both hands spread and held slightly more than shoulder width apart, bring the hands quickly together and align the five fingers

Fig. 22

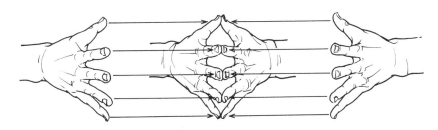

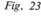
Fig. 23

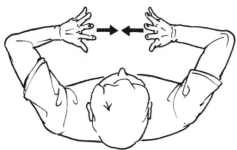

of one hand with the corresponding fingers of the other (Fig. 22 and 23). Repeat three times.

Unless the fingers of both hands are held slightly more than shoulder width apart, the exercise will fail to achieve its aim, which is to train the motor nerves and regulate the nerves in general. Though it seems easy, people whose motor nerves are dulled or whose auto-

nomic nervous system is unstable find this exercise difficult and should repeat it often to overcome the difficulty.

Performing it with closed eyes has a mentally unifying and concentrating effect. Stimulus from the fingers improves the functioning of the brain and helps maintain balance between the right and left lobes. In addition, it has a normalizing effect on the functioning of the internal organs.

● *Two-hand Stretching for the Little Fingers and Thumbs*

Placing the digital balls of the little finger and thumb of one hand firmly against those of the little finger and thumb of the other hand, bend the index, middle, and fourth fingers straight downward and bring the backs of those of one hand together with the backs of those of the other. Press the digital balls of little·fingers and thumbs together (Figs. 24–26). Hold this position ten seconds; repeat three times.

Repeated often, this shiatsu-stretching will strengthen and limber little fingers and thumbs. Furthermore, since the thumbs are related to the lungs and the little fingers to the heart, this exercise increases lung capacity and strengthens the heart.

Fig. 24

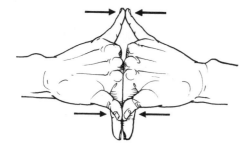

Fig. 26

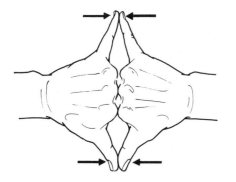

Fig. 25

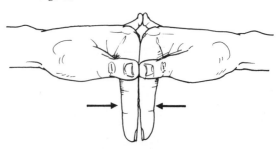

Incidentally, though probably with no conscious thought of the connection between the fingers and the internal organs, Japanese warriors of the past invariably practiced fencing moves that stretched the little fingers. The tensing of those fingers during downward swings of the practice sword was good training for the heart.

2. Cervical Region

Anterior Cervical Region

● *Shiatsu*

There are four shiatsu points on each side of
the anterior cervical region placed in a slanting
line from just above the clavicle to the region
immediately below the jaw (Figs. 1 and 2).
They lie on the sternocleidomastoid muscle in
the important zone where the common carotid
artery, which supplies blood to the face and
brain, passes.

   Since not only this, but also all shiatsu points
are related to the functioning of the heart and
blood circulation, as a rule, they are always
performed first on the left side. When the entire
left process has been completed, the operations
are performed on the right. Even when right
and left sides are treated simultaneously, the
order does not change. The first point on the
front of the neck is located in the carotid tri-
angle, where the common carotid artery divides
into the external carotid artery, which goes to
the face, and the internal carotid artery, which
goes to the brain. At this point, immediately
below the jaw, it is possible to feel the pulse by
light digital pressure.

   Shiatsu on the anterior cervical region begins

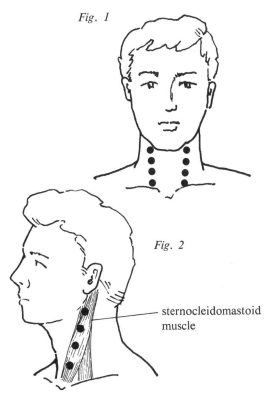

Fig. 1

Fig. 2

sternocleidomastoid
muscle

at point one and continues through point four
(Fig. 3). Pressure direction is toward the center
of the spinal column and the spinal process
(Fig. 4). Pressure should be light and applied

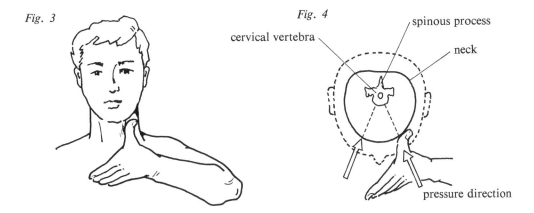

Fig. 3

Fig. 4

cervical vertebra

spinous process

neck

pressure direction

for only three seconds a time. The anterior cervical region is a sensitive area, and caution must be exercised to avoid excessive stimulation by applying too much pressure for too long.

Apply pressure to each point on the left side once and repeat the series three times. Then carry out the same process on the points on the right side.

Fig. 5

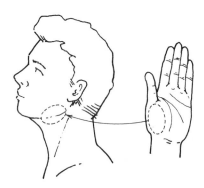

- *Stretching*

Pressing the bases of the thumbs, or the thenar, on the projection of the jaw immediately above points one, press both sides simultaneously rearward till the head is at an incline of about forty degrees. Hold this position for from five to ten seconds (Figs. 5–7). Repeat this stretching three times. In all cases, and especially in the case of the neck, pressure must be applied gradually, not suddenly. For this exercise to be effective, the upper body must be in a stable position; and the stretching must be concentrated in the anterior cervical region.

Fig. 6

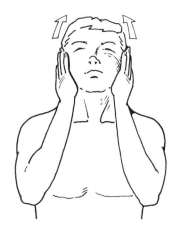

Fig. 7

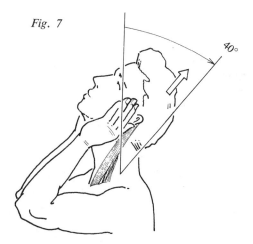

- *Stretching and Contracting*

This stretching and contracting exercise, which does not involve the hands, relies entirely on the automatic movement of the muscles. First, pull the chin in, thus relaxing the whole neck and especially the sternocleidomastoid muscle (Fig. 8-1). Next, thrusting the chin forward, incline the back of the head rearward on a slanting line (Fig. 8-2). Hold the head in this position for ten seconds to contract the sternocleidomastoid muscle. Then return the head to the relaxed position shown in Fig. 8-1. Finally, lower the neck from the base and stretch the back of the head diagonally upward. Hold this

Fig. 8

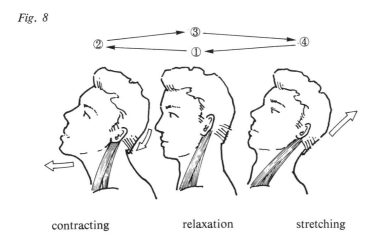

contracting   relaxation   stretching

stretched position for ten seconds (Figs. 8-3 and 4). Return the head to the relaxed position. Repeat the whole process three times.

Next, lie face-upward on a bed so that head and neck project beyond the edge. Stretch by lowering the head below the level of the top of the bed (Fig. 9-1). Hold this position for ten seconds. Contract the neck by raising the head (Fig. 9-2). Hold this position for ten seconds. Repeat the process three times.

Effects
Relieves myogenic torticollis, whiplash syndrome, insomnia, arteriosclerosis, eyestrain, chorditis, and hiccups. Regulates the secretion of thyroid hormones and prevents senile dementia.

contracting

Fig. 9

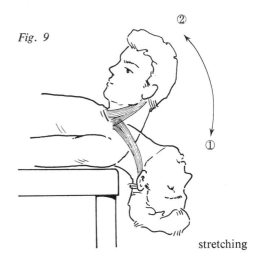

stretching

Lateral Cervical Region

Fig. 10

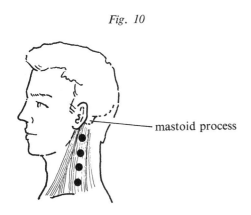

mastoid process

● *Shiatsu*
The shiatsu points for the lateral cervical region are located from the mastoid process to the suprascapular region. There are four such points on each side of the neck (Fig. 10) in the region where the neck muscles belonging to the sternocleidomastoid muscle group, the scalenus muscles, and the levator scapulae muscles are found.

Each of these points, beginning with number one, immediately below the mastoid process, is

Fig. 11

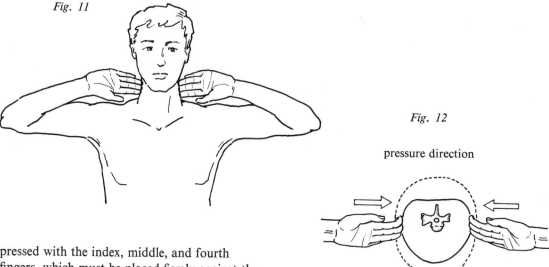

Fig. 12

pressure direction

pressed with the index, middle, and fourth fingers, which must be placed firmly against the neck. Pressure is applied on the right and left sides simultaneously and lasts for three seconds an application (Fig. 11). Pressure is applied directly to the neck from both sides (Fig. 12). To improve the effectiveness of this shiatsu, the elbows must be extended straight to the sides; and the upper body must be in a stable position. Repeat the process three times.

● *Stretching*
Interlocking the fingers of both hands, thumbs downward, press the thenars firmly against the neck and extend both elbows directly to the sides (Fig. 13). Remaining in this position, stretch the entire neck straight upward and hold this position for ten seconds (Fig. 14). Repeat three times. Next slowly bend the neck to the

left till the head is at an angle of fifty degrees. Holding this position, stretch the head diagonally upward (Fig. 15). The left hand serves only as support. The operation is performed with the left hand. When this stretching is complete, return the head to the original position; repeat three times. Then perform the same stretching exercise in the right direction (Fig. 16).

This stretching exercise limbers muscles in the lateral cervical zone and corrects faulty alignment (Fig. 17).

● *Stretching and Contracting*
Interlocking their fingers, place both hands on the top of the head and press downward to

Fig. 13

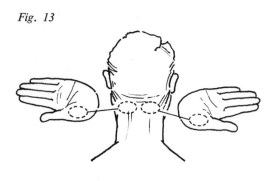

Fig. 14

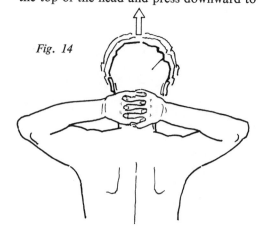

Fig. 15

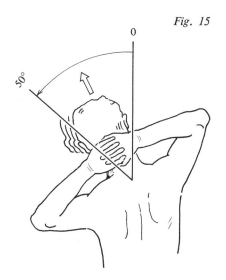

Fig. 16

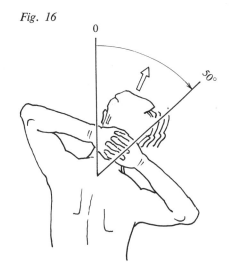

contract the neck (Fig. 18). As if in opposition to this pressure, tense the muscles of the right and left sides of the neck and maintain the contraction for ten seconds. Then, quickly removing the hands from the top of your head, stretch the neck upward (Fig. 19). Repeat the process three times. This exercise strengthens the neck muscle.

Effects
Brings relief from symptoms in the neck, shoulder, and arm muscles and the scalenus muscle group; relieves whiplash syndrome; and helps prevent arteriosclerosis, insomnia, headaches, stiff shoulders, ringing in the ears, and senile dementia.

Fig. 17

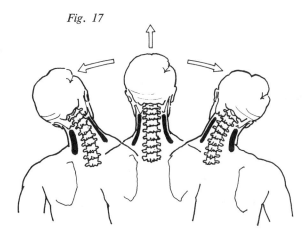

Fig. 18

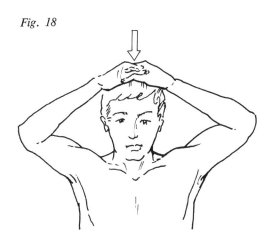

Fig. 19

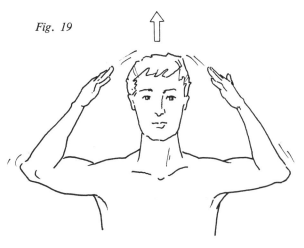

Region of the Medulla Oblongata

The region of the medulla oblongata is located at the boundary between the cervical and the occipital zones at the position of the occipital bone and the first cervical vertebra (Fig. 20). The medulla oblongata is in a depression at this region just large enough to be covered by

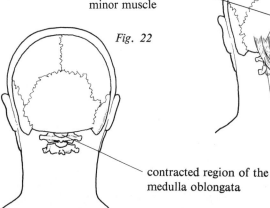

Fig. 20

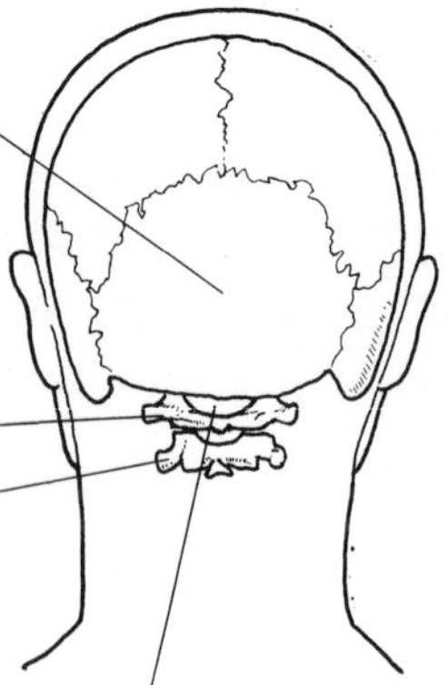

occipital bone

first cervical vertebra
second cervical vertebra

normal region of the medulla oblongata

Fig. 21

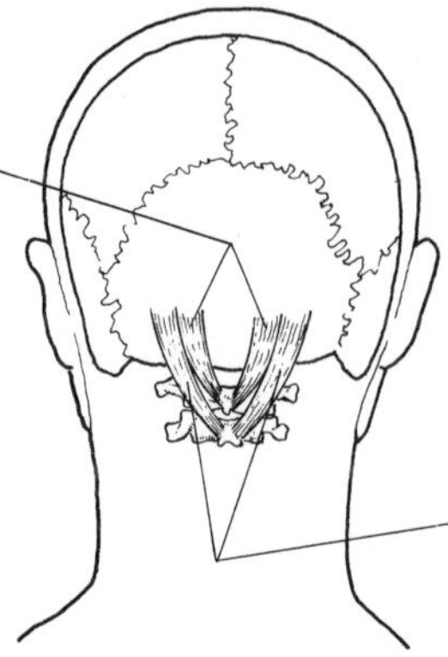

rectus capitis dorsalis minor muscle

Fig. 22

rectus capitis dorsalis major muscle

contracted region of the medulla oblongata

the fleshy ball of the thumb. The depression is bounded by the occipital bone and the right and left rectus capitis dorsalis minor muscles connecting with the first cervical vertebra and the left and right rectus capitis dorsalis major muscles, which connect with the second cervical vertebra. When these muscles stiffen, they narrow the depression and prevent shiatsu pressure from reaching the medulla oblongata (Figs. 21 and 22). In such cases, it is important to limber these muscles by applying pressure with the index, middle, and fourth fingers to the surrounding muscles and thus opening the interstice between the occipital bone and the first cervical vertebra and allowing shiatsu pressure to penetrate to the medulla oblongata (Figs. 23 and 24).

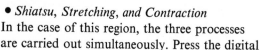

Fig. 23 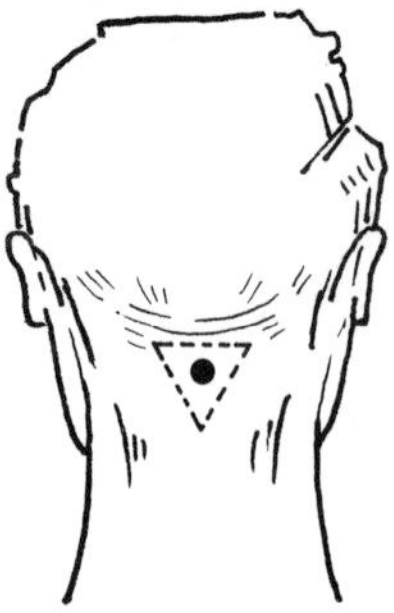 *Fig. 24*

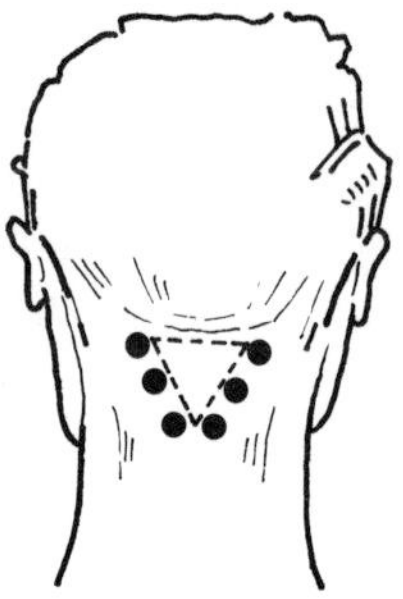

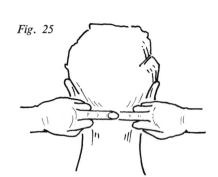

Fig. 25

● *Shiatsu, Stretching, and Contraction*
In the case of this region, the three processes are carried out simultaneously. Press the digital

ball of the left middle finger over the medulla oblongata and put the digital ball of the right middle finger on top of it. Extending both elbows directly to the sides, apply pressure on a line crossing between the eyebrows. At the same time, stretch the medulla oblongata by slowly inclining the head forward thirty degrees (Figs. 25–27-1 and 2). Return the head to the normal position. Then, applying pressure to the medulla oblongata, incline it rearward thirty degrees (Figs. 27-2 and 3). This contracts the medulla oblongata. Hold the position for ten seconds, then repeat the entire process three times.

Effects
There is good foundation for the old tradition that tapping the area of the medulla oblongata

or pulling the hair in that region stops nose-bleed. Stimulating the medulla oblongata, which is a center of vasoconstriction in this area, brings on constriction of the blood vessels and consequent cessation of hemorrhage. The stimulus of tapping, however, is too great; and it is much better to apply steady, gently pressure. In addition, these exercises halt nose-bleed, stimulate cerebral functioning, stimulate the pituitary gland, and regulate its hormone secretion. In addition, they bring relief from insomnia, whiplash syndrome, headaches, heaviness of the head, and menopause symptoms and prevent senile dementia.

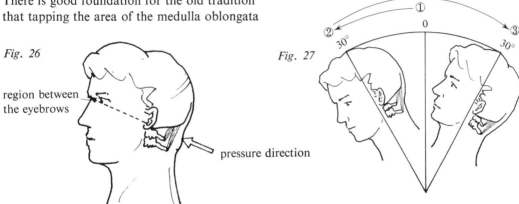

Fig. 26

region between the eyebrows

pressure direction

Fig. 27

Posterior Cervical Region

● *Shiatsu*
In this region, shiatsu pressure is applied to two rows of four points beginning with the first, at the height of the medulla oblongata, and continuing to the fourth at the base of the neck (Fig. 28). Applied simultaneously with the index, middle, and fourth fingers of both hands, pressure, which is directed toward the center of the face, lasts for three seconds per application on each point (Figs. 29 and 30). The whole series is repeated three times. This will limber the posterior cervical muscles (trapezius, splenius cervicis, and semispinalis capitis).

Fig. 28

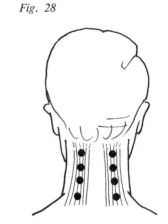

Fig. 29

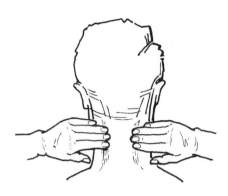

Fig. 30

central facial region

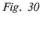

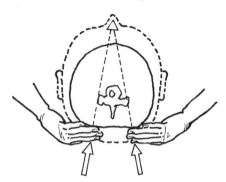

pressure direction

● *Stretching*

As was done in stretching for the lateral cervical region, interlock the fingers of both hands and press the thenars of both hands immediately below the occipital region. Press the full palms of both hands against the posterior cervical zone. From this relaxed posture, gradually lean the head forward in a bowing motion to stretch (Figs. 31 and 32). Hold the stretched position ten seconds and repeat the exercise three times.

● *Stretching and Contracting*

After stretching, first return to the normal up-right position then contract the muscles of the posterior cervical region by leaning the head rearward (Figs. 33 and 34). Hold this position ten seconds, return to the normal position, stretch by leaning forward and holding the position for ten seconds, and repeat the series three times.

Effects

Brings relief from occipital neuralgia, heaviness and pain in the head, migraine, whiplash syndrome, arteriosclerosis, insomnia, and dizziness and helps prevent senile dementia.

Fig. 31

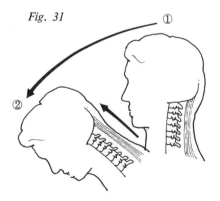

Fig. 32

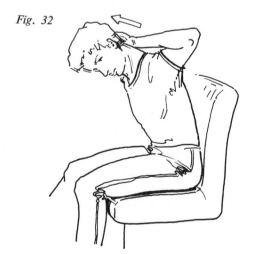

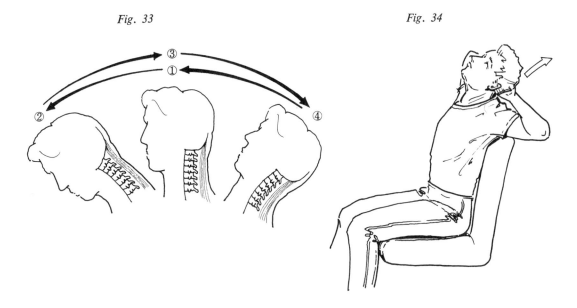

Fig. 33   Fig. 34

3. Scapular Region and Upper Limbs

Suprascapular Region

● *Shiatsu*

Shiatsu points for the shoulder are on the shoulder blade adjacent to the lowest of the four lateral cervical points (Figs. 1 and 2) in the locations of the trapezius, levator scapulae, and supraspinatus muscles (Figs. 3 and 4). Shiatsu pressure, applied with the digital balls of the index, middle, and fourth fingers of the right hand is strong and should be directed to the center of the trunk at the height of the diaphragm (Figs. 5 and 6). Each application

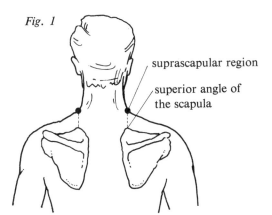

Fig. 1

suprascapular region

superior angle of the scapula

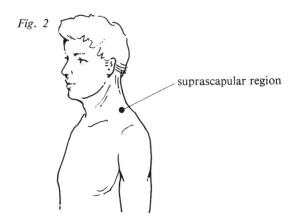

Fig. 2

suprascapular region

38

Fig. 3

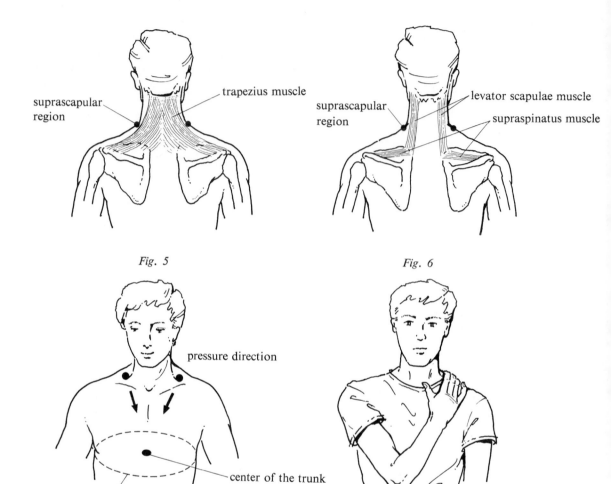

suprascapular region

trapezius muscle

Fig. 4

suprascapular region

levator scapulae muscle

supraspinatus muscle

Fig. 5

pressure direction

center of the trunk

height of the diaphragm

Fig. 6

should last for five seconds. Repeat three times. Then apply pressure in the same way to the suprascapular point on the right shoulder with the index, middle, and fourth fingers of the left hand.

The position at which the suprascapular point is located must support the weight of the neck and head. This requires tensing of the muscle groups in the region, and this in turn is what tends to cause stiff shoulders (Fig. 7).

Fig. 7

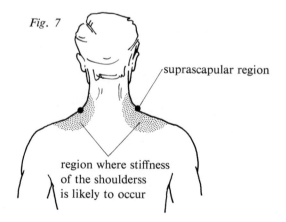

suprascapular region

region where stiffness of the shoulderss is likely to occur

Fig. 8

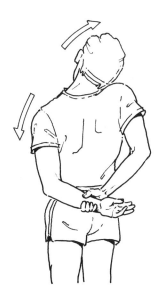

● Stretching

To stretch the shoulder region, incline the head to the right. From behind your back, grip your left wrist in your right hand and pull it downward. Stretch this way for ten seconds (Fig. 8). This thoroughly stretches the cervical and scapular zones and relaxes their muscle groups. Return your head to the normal position. Repeat three times. Then perform the same exercise on the left side.

Fig. 9

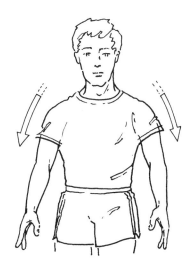

● Stretching and Contracting

Allow both arms to descend naturally slightly away from the body. Maintaining this position, pull both arms downward (Fig. 9). Hold this stretched position for ten seconds. Then, without altering the positions of your arms, raise both shoulders as high as possible in a shrugging motion to contract the muscles (Fig. 10). Hold this for five seconds. Repeat the stretching and contracting three times.

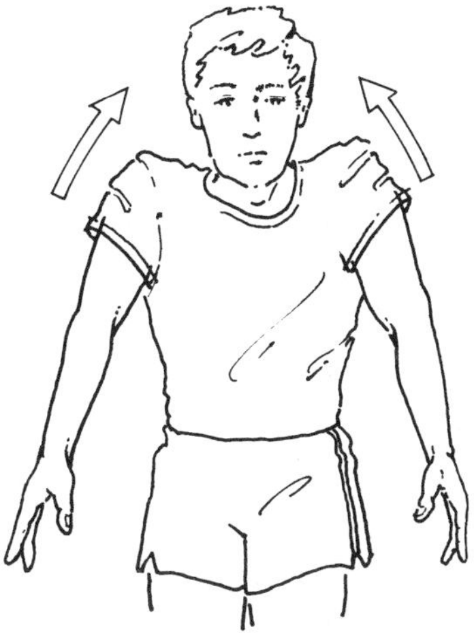

Effects

In addition to stiff shoulders caused by fatigue, this exercise helps cure shoulder pathological-reflex stiffness caused by disorders in the internal organs. Such stiffness is brought on by what is called cutaneovisceral reflexes. To cure it, shiatsu pressure applied to the surface of the body stimulates reflex action in and thereby regulates the functioning of the internal organs.

- Left suprascapular region: heart, stomach, pancreas, left kidney, descending colon, and sigmoid colon
- Right suprascapular region: liver, gallbladder, right kidney, and ascending colon

Fig. 10

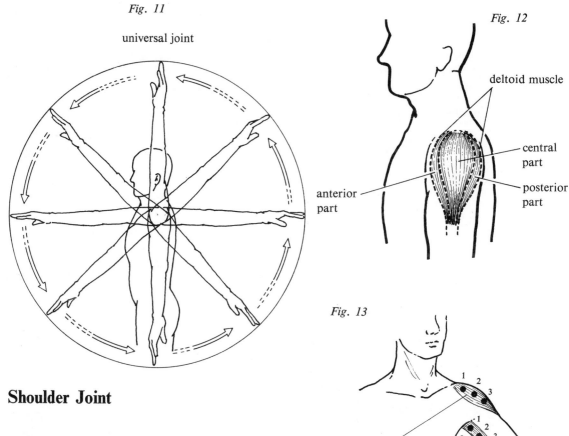

Fig. 11

universal joint

Fig. 12

deltoid muscle

central part

posterior part

anterior part

Fig. 13

anterior deltoid region

coracobrachial muscle

Shoulder Joint

● *Shiatsu*

The joint between the humerus and the scapula, called a universal joint, has the widest range of motion of any joint in the body (Fig. 11). Among the many muscles attached to it is the deltoid muscle, which accounts from the rounded appearance of the shoulders (Fig. 12). Contraction of the anterior part of the deltoid muscle and of the coracobrachial muscle accounts for flexion and elevation of the upper arm (Fig. 13). Shiatsu on the deltoid muscle is applied first to the three points in the anterior deltoid region of the left shoulder with the thumb of the right hand. The tip of the thumb is pointed upward; and pressure is applied, for three seconds, downward. For the coracobrachial muscle, it is applied to the four points in the axillary region of the left arm with the thumb, in the same fashion. Each application lasts for three seconds. The procedures

for both are then repeated on the right arm. (Below, explanations are given for the left side only, but remember, ALL SHIATSU APPLICATIONS MUST BE REPEATED ON THE RIGHT SIDE.)

Abduction of the upper arm is performed by the central region of the deltoid and by the supraspinatus muscles (Figs. 14 and 16). Shiatsu is applied to the three points leading from the left suprascapular region and across the supraspinatus muscle with the index, middle, and fourth fingers of the right hand. Similar pressure is then applied to the points of the central region of the deltoid muscle. Repeat each application three times and then perform

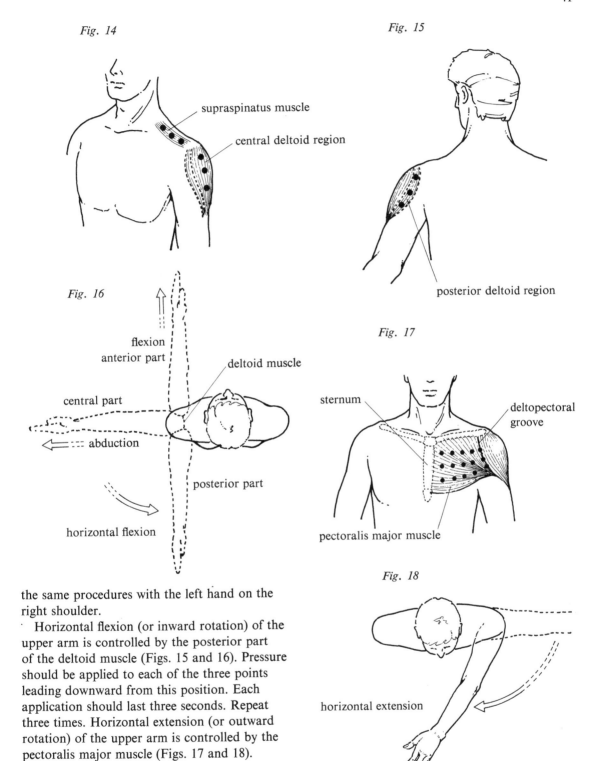

Fig. 14

supraspinatus muscle

central deltoid region

Fig. 15

posterior deltoid region

Fig. 16

flexion
anterior part

deltoid muscle

central part

abduction

posterior part

horizontal flexion

Fig. 17

sternum

deltopectoral
groove

pectoralis major muscle

Fig. 18

horizontal extension

the same procedures with the left hand on the right shoulder.

Horizontal flexion (or inward rotation) of the upper arm is controlled by the posterior part of the deltoid muscle (Figs. 15 and 16). Pressure should be applied to each of the three points leading downward from this position. Each application should last three seconds. Repeat three times. Horizontal extension (or outward rotation) of the upper arm is controlled by the pectoralis major muscle (Figs. 17 and 18). Shiatsu for it is performed first with the right thumb on the three points descending diagonally on the deltopectoral groove. Application lasts for three seconds and is repeated three times. Next pressure is applied to three horizontal rows of four points each. The first row begins at the sternum and, running immediately below the clavicle, extends to the deltopectoral groove. Press each point for three seconds with the thumb of the right hand; repeat three times. The other two rows are located below this first one in the spaces between each member of two pairs of ribs. Pressure on all these points regulates the performance of the deltoid and pectoralis major muscles.

Internal rotation of the shoulder joint—extending the arm straight to the side at shoulder

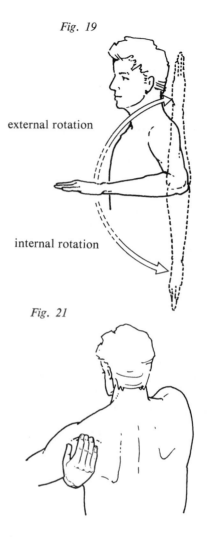

Fig. 19

external rotation

internal rotation

Fig. 20

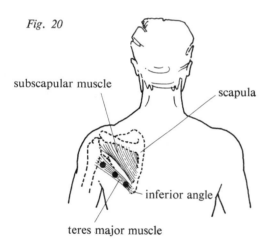

subscapular muscle

scapula

inferior angle

teres major muscle

Fig. 21

height then, maintaining the same height, bringing the elbow ninety degrees inward (Fig. 19)—is controlled by the subscapular and the teres major muscles (Fig. 20). Shiatsu is applied on a diagonally descending line of three points on the teres major muscle, which is located below the scapula. To carry it out, bring your right hand around to your back under your left armpit. With its index, middle, and fourth fingers, press each of the points shown for three seconds; repeat six times (Fig. 21). Press the teres major muscle thoroughly, since the subscapular muscle is located beneath it and cannot be pressed directly.

External rotation, the reverse of internal

rotation, is controlled by the infraspinatus and teres minor muscles (Fig. 22). To perform shiatsu on these muscles, just as in the preceding application, bring your right hand around to your back under your left armpit. Place its index, middle, and fourth fingers at the head of the humerus. Three points are located on the infraspinatus muscle, which runs under the spine of the scapula. Press each of these points three times for three seconds each time (Fig. 23). Then, in the same way, press each of the three points on the teres minor muscle three times for three seconds each. The condition known as scapulohumeral periarthritis, which occurs in middle age, hinders

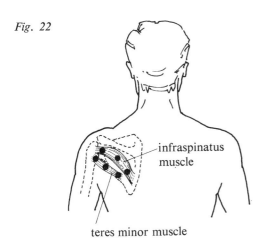

Fig. 22

infraspinatus
muscle

teres minor muscle

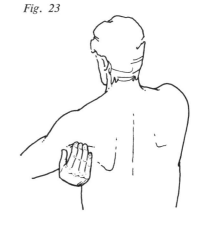

Fig. 23

external rotation and makes it difficult to do such things as hold a comb in the right hand and comb the hair from the temporal to the occipital zone.

● *Stretching*
Thrust both shoulders simultaneously forward as far as possible (Fig. 24). Hold this position for five seconds. Pull both shoulders backward simultaneously as far as possible. Hold this

position for five seconds. Repeat three times. Next roll both shoulders forward simultaneously as wide as possible (Fig. 25). Repeat five times. Then roll them backward in a similar fashion. Repeat five times.

Finally perform ultra-stretching of the shoulders in this way. Stretch your left arm straight up with palm turned rearward and your right arm straight down with palm turned rearward (Fig. 26). Next bend your left forearm down

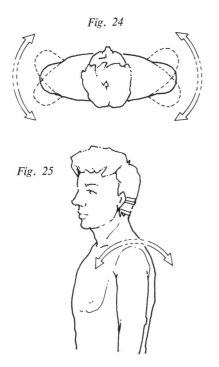

Fig. 24

Fig. 25

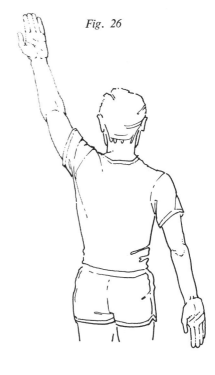

Fig. 26

Fig. 27

Fig. 28

external rotation

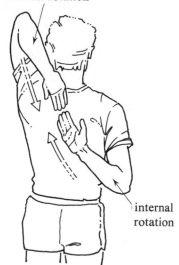

internal
rotation

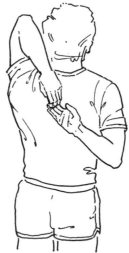

Fig. 29

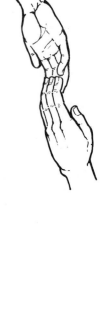

Fig. 30

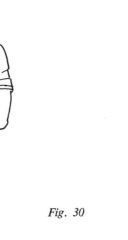

and your right forearm up and bring the tips of
the fingers of both hands as close together as
possible (Figs. 27 and 28). Interlock them if
you can (Figs. 29 and 30). This exercise simultaneously rotates the left arm out and the right
arm in. Repeat with the arms in reversed relations.

Effects
Brings relief from stiffness of the shoulders and
scapulohumeral periarthritis.

Upper Arm

As in the preceding section, explanation is given
for shiatsu and stretching on the left side only.
When this has been completed, the same procedures should be performed on the right side.

● *Shiatsu*
The inner muscle group in the upper arm is
responsible for flexing and the outer muscle
group for extending of the elbow.

Six shiatsu points are located along the inner
side of the left upper arm from the armpit
(axilla) to the cubital fossa on the biceps brachii
and the brachial muscles (Fig. 31). With the
thumb of the right hand, press each of these
points three times for three seconds each time
(Fig. 32).

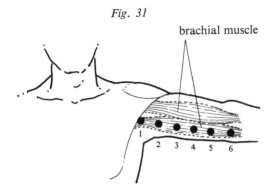

Fig. 31

brachial muscle

1 2 3 4 5 6

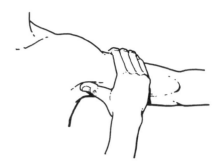

Fig. 32

Fig. 33

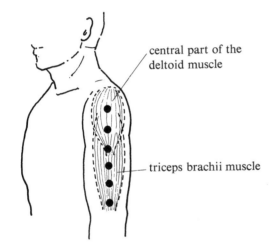

central part of the deltoid muscle

triceps brachii muscle

On the outer side of the upper arm are six shiatsu points located from the central part of the deltoid muscle along the triceps brachii muscle and to the elbow (Fig. 33). Press each three times with the thumb of the right hand for three seconds each (Fig. 34).

● *Stretching*
Gripping the left elbow in the right hand and pulling down simultaneously stretch the biceps and triceps brachii muscles (Fig. 35). The arm naturally stretches without tensing. Pull down for five seconds and then relax the right hand and allow the arm to return to normal position. Repeat three times.

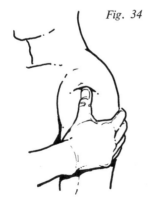

Fig. 34

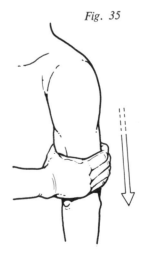

Fig. 35

Elbow

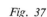
Fig. 36

● *Shiatsu*

The left arm is allowed to hang naturally with the back of the hand turned out, and shiatsu is applied from the outside of the elbow joint. The three shiatsu points are located on a diagonal downward line starting at the olecranon (Fig. 36). With the thumb of the right hand, turned up, and the other four fingers wrapped around the elbow for support, press each of these points three times for three seconds each time (Fig. 37).

Shiatsu on the cubital fossa is applied on three points on a horizontal line starting on the inner side and moving outward (Fig. 38). Press each of these points with the thumb of

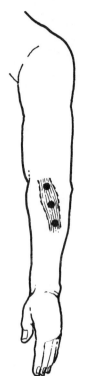

Fig. 37

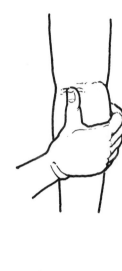

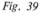
Fig. 38

Fig. 39

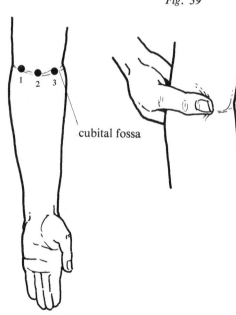

cubital fossa

Fig. 40

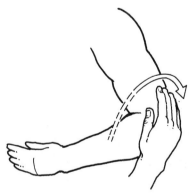

the right hand (pointed outward) three times for three seconds each time (Fig. 39).

Finally, bending the left elbow, wrap the right palm around the olecranon and rotate it ten times in the clockwise direction (Fig. 40).

Each rotation should last one second. Repeat the process three times.

● *Stretching*

Extend the left arm, with the palm up. Grip

its wrist—thumb underside and four fingers wrapped around the top—with the right hand and pull straight, with a slight downward inclination. Hold the stretched position ten seconds then gradually relax the right-hand pull (Fig. 41). Repeat three times.

Fig. 41

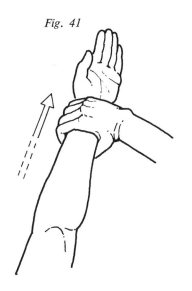

Forearm

● *Shiatsu*

Outstretch the left arm with the palm turned upward. There are three rows of eight shiatsu points each on the inner side of the forearm (Fig. 42). They lead from immediately below the cubital fossa toward the wrist. With the thumb of the right hand (directed toward the wrist) and with the other four fingers wrapped behind the arm for support, press each of these points three times for three seconds each time. Pressure should be directed slightly toward the wrist (Fig. 43).

For shiatsu on the outer side of the forearm, naturally extend the left arm, with the back of the hand turned outward. Pressure is applied to the extensor muscle group, the mound extending from the middle finger to the elbow (Fig. 44). The first point is at the attachment of the extensor digitorum communis muscle, which can be located by bending the four fingers upward and downward and thus causing the muscle to move visibly. Strong pressure on this point affects the radial nerve above the radia and causes pain. With the right thumb (pointed toward the elbow) and with the other

Fig. 42

cubital fossa *Fig. 43*

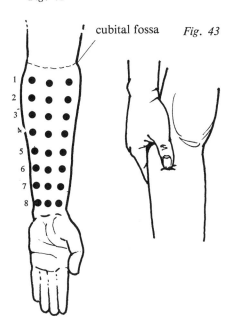

Fig. 44

Fig. 45

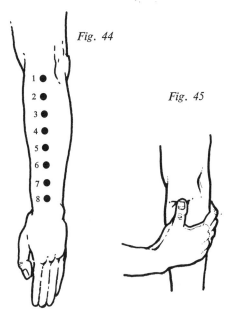

four fingers wrapped around the arm for support, press each of the eight points running from the attachment of the extensor digitorum communis to the wrist three times for three seconds each time (Fig. 45).

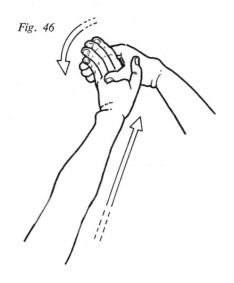

Fig. 46

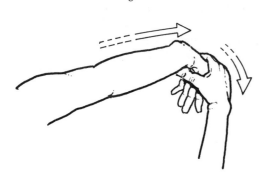

Fig. 47

● *Stretching*

With the palm turned downward, extend the left forearm. With the right thumb placed against the dorsal bases of the fingers and the other four fingers against the palmar bases for support, stretch the flexor muscle group by bending the fingers backward (dorsiflexion; Fig. 46). Hold the bent position for ten seconds then release. Repeat three times.

To stretch the outer side of the forearm, leave the arm in the same position, with the palm turned down, place the four fingers of the right hand against the dorsal surface of the left wrist and the right thumb against the palmar surface of the wrist for support and bend the hand fully inward (Fig. 47). This stretches the extensor muscle group. Hold the bent position for ten seconds and repeat three times.

Wrist and Fingers

Shiatsu and stretching for the fingers are performed as explained in the section on Finger Warm-up. It is permissible to perform these exercises before treating the whole or other parts of the body.

● *Stretching the Upper Limbs*

With the fingers of both hands interlocked, extend both arms straight forward. Rotate the interlocked hands to the left (Figs. 48 and 49),

Fig. 48

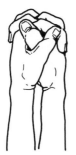

Fig. 49

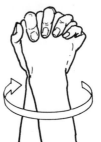

Fig. 50

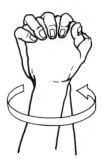

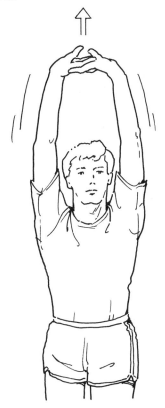

Fig. 51

with the wrists as the fulcrum of the motion. This simultaneously causes pronation of the right and supination of the left hand. Then rotate them to the right, causing supination of the right and pronation of the left hand (Fig. 50). Each rotation should last five seconds. Rotate first to the left then to the right and repeat the series three times.

Extend both arms directly overhead with the palms turned up, the fingers of both hands interlocked, and stretch upward (Fig. 51). Relax all of the body except the arms and do not allow it to be included in the stretch. Each pull should last for ten seconds; repeat three times.

With the fingers still interlocked, lower both arms till they are extended horizontally forward. Stretch them forward in this position (Fig. 52). Hold the stretch for ten seconds and repeat three times.

Then, with fingers interlocked and turned inward, extend both hands rearward, behind your back, and bring them as nearly straight and as close to the horizontal position as possible. Hold the stretch for ten seconds and repeat three times (Fig. 53).

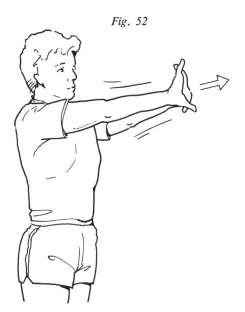

Fig. 52

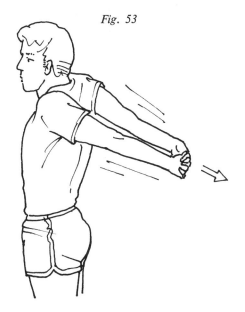

Fig. 53

Effects of Shiatsu and Stretching of the Upper Limbs

Relief from brachial neuralgia, pain in the elbow joint, so-called tennis elbow, writer's cramp, Raynaud's disease, chilling of the fingers, paralysis of the upper limbs, and numbness in the hand.

∗ Cutaneovisceral Reflexes

Disorders in internal organs and vessels reflect in hardness or stiffness in the places on the hands where cutaneovisceral reflexes manifest themselves. Consequently, shiatsu applied to these points stimulates reflexes in the organs and thus regulates their functioning.

Right hand (Fig. 54)
    Thumb—lungs
    Index finger—liver, gallbladder, eyes
    Middle finger—large and small intestines
    Fourth and little fingers—heart, kidneys, urinary bladder
    Palmar center—diaphragm
Left hand (Fig. 55)
    Thumb—lungs
    Index finger—stomach, pancreas, eyes
    Middle finger—large and small intestines
    Fourth and little fingers—heart, kidneys, urinary bladder
    Palmar center—diaphragm

Fig. 54

Fig. 55

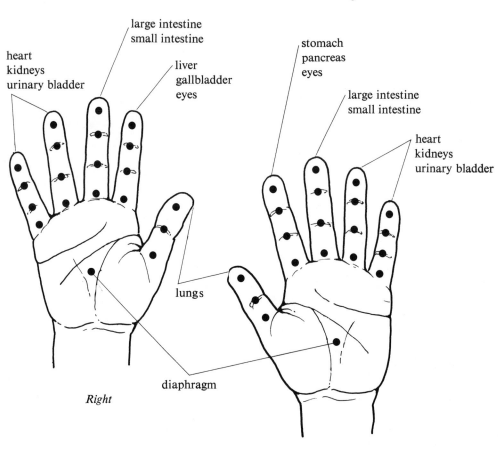

heart
kidneys
urinary bladder

large intestine
small intestine

liver
gallbladder
eyes

stomach
pancreas
eyes

large intestine
small intestine

heart
kidneys
urinary bladder

lungs

diaphragm

Right

Left

4. Lower Limbs

The explanations are given for the left side only, though, of course, the identical treatment must be applied to the right side as well.

Anterior Thigh Region

● *Shiatsu*

Shiatsu for the anterior left thigh begins at the inguinal region, in the center of the thigh at the point where the leg joins the trunk (Figs. 1 and 2). Since this is the area through which the femoral artery and femoral nerve pass, pressure on it stimulates both circulation and nerve functioning. Applied with the thenar of the left hand, pressure is directed inward and lasts for five seconds (Fig. 3). Repeat three times.

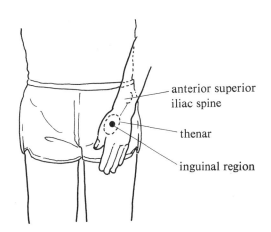

Fig. 1

anterior superior iliac spine

thenar

inguinal region

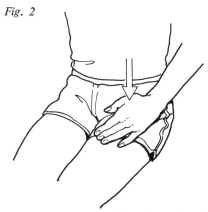

Fig. 2

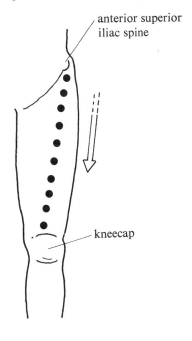

Fig. 3

anterior superior iliac spine

kneecap

Next apply pressure three times for three seconds each application to the ten points leading from directly below the anterior superior iliac spine, located diagonally above the inguinal region, along the quadriceps femoris muscle almost to the knee (Fig. 2). The pressure is applied with both thumbs, the right on top of the left, and with the four fingers of each hand wrapped around the thigh for support (Figs. **4** and **5**). The quadriceps femoris extends the knee and raises the lower leg.

Fig. 4

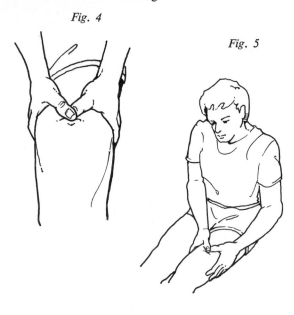

Fig. 5

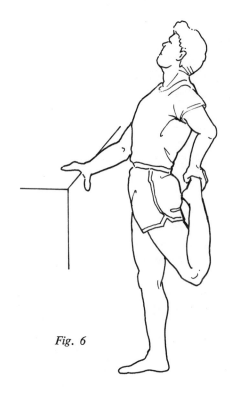

Fig. 6

● *Stretching*
Stretch the quadriceps femoris muscle by standing straight, putting the right hand on a table or other object of similar height for support, and raising your left leg to the rear until the heel comes in close contact with the buttock. Then, gripping the bases of the toes of the left foot with the thumb and four fingers of the left hand, pull upward (Fig. 6). Hold for ten seconds then lower the leg to its normal position. Lightly relax before repeating. Perform the stretch three times.

Medial Region of the Thigh

Fig. 7

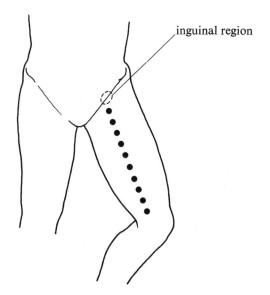

inguinal region

● *Shiatsu*
For treatment of the medial side of the thigh, bend the left knee and turn it outward. With thumb on thumb (left thumb on the bottom), apply pressure to each of the ten points running along the center line of the medial surface of

the thigh, beginning from immediately below the inguinal region and continuing almost to the knee (Fig. 7). Pressure is applied for three seconds to each point and is repeated three times. This shiatsu is for the adductor muscle group, which draws the medial side of the thigh inward.

● *Stretching*
Sitting on the floor, bring the soles of the feet together and pull the heels as far inward as possible. With one hand on each of the thighs, near the knees, press firmly and slowly downward to bring the thighs close to the floor (Fig. 8). Hold this position for ten seconds then relax pressure. Repeat three times.

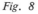
Fig. 8

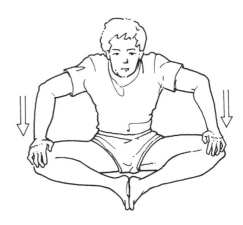

Hip Joint

● *Shiatsu*
The projection about ten centimeters diagonally below the anterior superior iliac spine, on the center line of the lateral side of the thigh is the greater trochanter of the femur (Figs. 9 and 10). Shiatsu for the hip joint begins at that point. Pressing the palm of the left hand against

the greater trochanter, bend and raise the left knee to the height of the hip joint. Remaining in this position, swing the lower leg (from the knee downward) to the right and the left (Fig. 11), thus rotating the hip joint inward and outward. If there is stiffness or other irregularity in the hip joint, this inward-outward rotation will not be smooth.

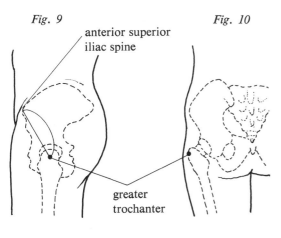

Fig. 9   *Fig. 10*

anterior superior iliac spine

greater trochanter

left lateral region   left posterior region

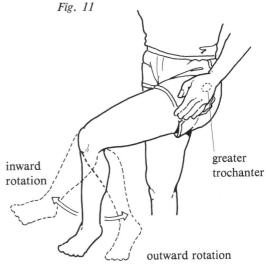

Fig. 11

inward rotation

greater trochanter

outward rotation

Fig. 12

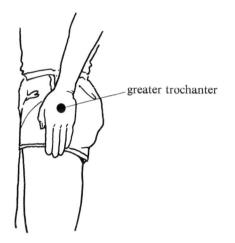

greater trochanter

A great many muscles are attached at the greater trochanter. To treat them, after applying pressure to the greater trochanter itself three times for five seconds each, with the left thumb, apply pressure to each of the six points around it (Figs. 12 and 13). Apply pressure, moving in a counterclockwise direction: three applications lasting three seconds each.

Finally apply pressure, from above and directed diagonally downward toward the hip joint, to the three points on the gluteus medius muscle and the four points on the gluteus maximus muscle: three applications, each lasting three seconds, on each point (Fig. 14).

● *Stretching*

Standing turned sideways with the right hand resting on a table or the wall, raise your left leg as high as possible in front of you. Then, slowly make a circle with your left foot, swinging it first from the front to the side and then from the side to the rear (Fig. 15). Next return it to the front and lower it to the floor. The full stretch should take five seconds. Repeat it three times. The leg must be raised as high as possible, and the knee must not bend during

Fig. 13

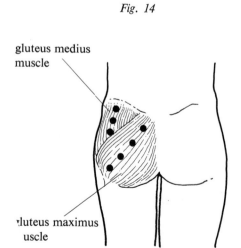

greater trochanter

Fig. 14

gluteus medius muscle

ˈluteus maximus uscle

Fig. 15

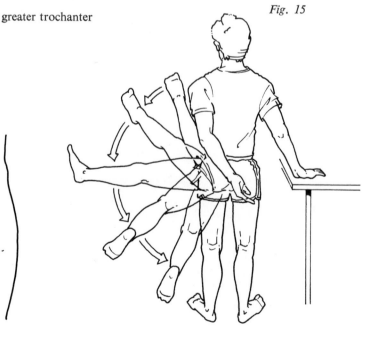

the rearward swing. When this is finished, perform a similar swing, starting from the rear and moving forward; this too should take five seconds and should be repeated three times.

Lateral Region of the Thigh

• *Shiatsu*
Seated on the floor with both legs outstretched, apply pressure to the ten points, on the center line of the outer side of the thigh beginning immediately below the greater trochanter (Fig. 16). Pressure should be applied with both thumbs, held tip to tip but not overlapped, and with the four fingers of each hand outspread or wrapped around the leg for support (Fig. 17). The pressure should be directed toward the center of the thigh. Each application should last for three seconds; repeat three times. This treatment is for the tensor fasciae latae muscles and the iliotibial ligament.

• *Stretching*
Sitting in a chair, cross your legs, left thigh on right thigh. Place the interlocked fingers of both hands against the outer side of the left knee. Pull to the right to stretch the left thigh (Fig. 18). Hold for ten seconds and repeat three times.

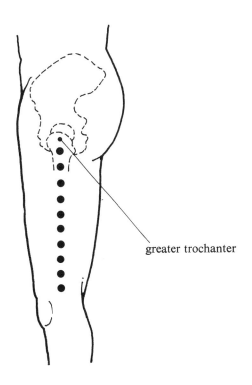

Fig. 16

greater trochanter

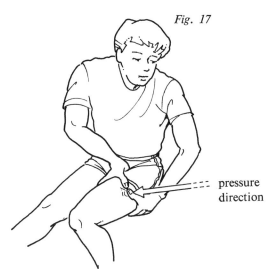

Fig. 17

pressure direction

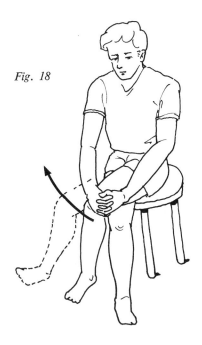

Fig. 18

Knee

• *Shiatsu*

Above the knee and covering the kneecap, or patella, is the tendon of the quadriceps femoris muscle. Below the kneecap, it attaches with the patellar ligament (Fig. 19). These muscles and ligament extend the knee and move the lower leg. When fatigue accumulates there, the knee becomes stiff; and bending it grows painful. Thorough shiatsu limbers the knee and stimulates the secretion of the synovial fluid needed for smooth knee action.

To perform this shiatsu, sit on the floor with both legs outstretched to the front. Bend the left knee enough to raise it slightly from the floor. With both thumbs, tip to tip but not overlapped, and with the four fingers of both hands wrapped around the popliteal fossa for support, apply pressure to the points around the knee joint, beginning with the three below the knee and working from outside inward (Figs. 20 and 21). Press each point for three seconds. Then apply pressure to the three points above the knee, once again moving from outside inward. Repeat these two sets of pressure applications three times.

Next, with the fingers held together, place the left palm above the knee. Put the right hand on top of the left (Fig. 22) and execute circular palmar pressure inward and outward ten times each at a rate of one rotation per

Fig. 19

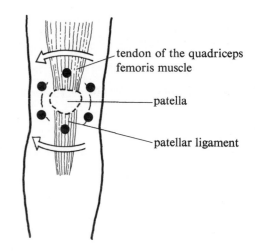

tendon of the quadriceps femoris muscle

patella

patellar ligament

Fig. 20

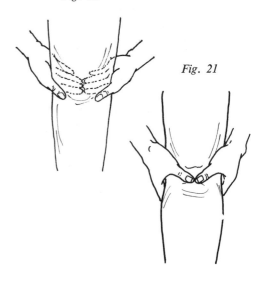

Fig. 21

Fig. 22

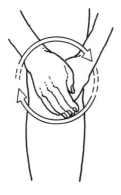

second. It is important to avoid applying strong pressure and to rotate the palm lightly as if it were drawing the knee upward to itself.

• *Stretching*

To stretch the knee, stand on your right foot and bend your left knee. Hold your left ankle in your left hand and pull until your left heel touches your left buttock. Then simultaneously press rearward on your left knee with your right hand and pull your left ankle with your left hand (Fig. 23). Hold ten seconds and repeat three times.

Slightly Lateral Anterior Region of the Lower Legs

● *Shiatsu*

Sit either on the floor with legs outstretched forward or in a chair. In the latter instance, place another chair in front of you and put your left foot in its seat. Turning the left knee slightly inward, bring it toward the right knee, which serves as a support, and turn the lateral anterior region of the lower leg upward (Figs. 24 and 25). The first shiatsu point in this region

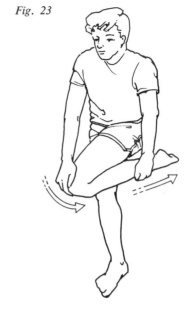

Fig. 23

is located about three centimeters below the point of projection of the tibia immediately below the knee (Fig. 26). With both thumbs, the left one on the bottom, and with the fingers of the hands wrapped around the leg for support, press firmly on this point for five seconds. The pressure is directed toward the tibia. Repeat three times. Since this affects the deep

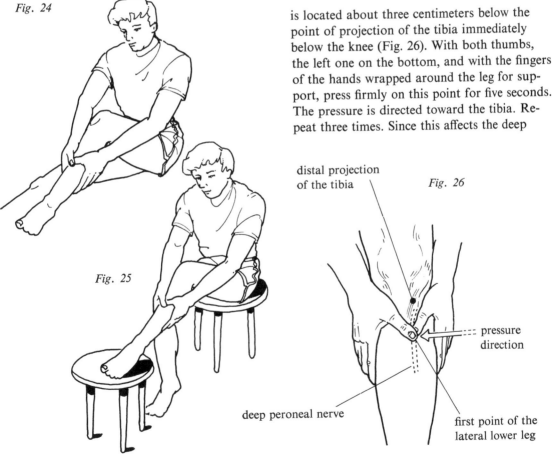

Fig. 24

Fig. 25

distal projection of the tibia

Fig. 26

pressure direction

deep peroneal nerve

first point of the lateral lower leg

Fig. 27

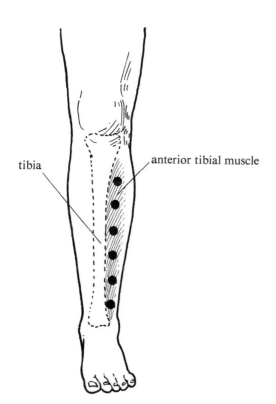

tibia

anterior tibial muscle

peroneal nerve, it will cause sharp pain. Continue applying pressure on the remaining five points between this one and the ankle (Fig. 27). Each application lasts three seconds. Repeat three times.

Ankle, Dorsal Surface of the Foot, and Toes

● *Shiatsu*

The front part of the ankle is the region through which pass the tendons of the extensor muscle group, which are attached to the toes. Thorough shiatsu on it limbers the ankle, removes stiffness, and facilitates extension of the toes. Pressure is applied with both thumbs, held tip to tip but not overlapping. The four fingers of each hand are wrapped around the foot for support. Working from the lateral malleolus on the outer side toward the medial malleolus on the inner side, press each of the three points for three seconds (Fig. 28 and 29). Repeat three times.

Shiatsu on the dorsal surface of the foot is performed on the four points between the metatarsal bones between the big and second toes, on the four between the second and third toes, on the four between the third and

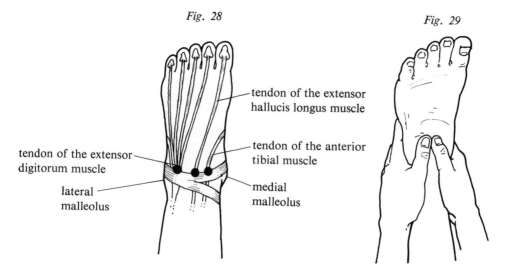

Fig. 28

Fig. 29

tendon of the extensor hallucis longus muscle

tendon of the anterior tibial muscle

tendon of the extensor digitorum muscle

lateral malleolus

medial malleolus

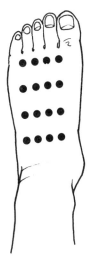

Fig. 30

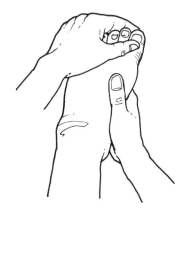

Fig. 31

fourth toes, and on the four between the fourth
and little toes (Fig. 30). The rows of points
begin at the bases of the toes. To treat them,
wrap the thumb and fingers of the left hand
around the left toes as shown in Fig. 31. Apply
pressure with the right thumb, beginning at
the bases of the toes and moving toward the
ankle. Each pressure application should last
for three seconds. Treatment of each of the
four series of points should be repeated three
times.

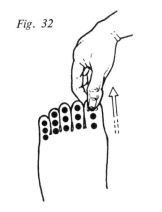

Fig. 32

Each of the left toes is gripped between the
right thumb and index finger, which are used to
apply pressure (Fig. 32). Three points on each
toe are on a line beginning at the base and
moving toward the tip. After pressure has been
applied for three seconds to each point, at the
third point, which is located at the tip of the
toe, pull straight forward for one second. Apply
pressure to all fifteen points without stopping
and repeat the entire series of fifteen three
times.

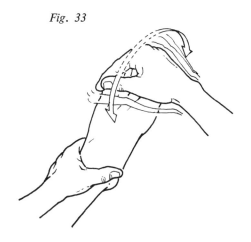

Fig. 33

Finally, supporting the left ankle with the
left hand, place the palm of the right hand on
the tips of the toes and rhythmically move all
the toes forward and backward to cause
plantarflexion and dorsiflexion of the joints
(Fig. 33).

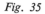

Fig. 34

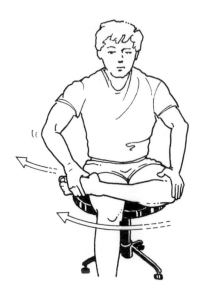

Fig. 35

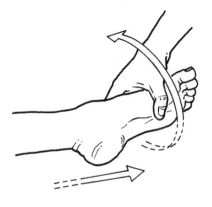

Fig. 36

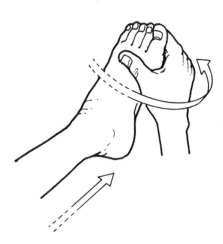

Fig. 37

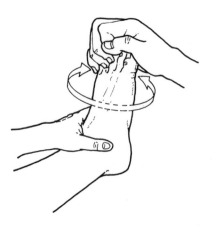

● *Stretching*

Sitting either in a chair or on the floor with both legs outstretched forward, bend the left leg and bring the lateral side of the left thigh on top of the right knee. The sole of the left foot is turned inward. With the left hand against the right knee for support, grip the left foot firmly with the right hand (thumb on the sole and fingers on the dorsal surface) and pull (Fig. 34). This one operation stretches ankle, dorsal surface of the foot, and lower leg at the same time. Hold the pull for ten seconds and repeat three times.

Next perform inversion stretching by remaining in the same posture and rotating the sole of the foot inward (Fig. 35). The inversion should take ten seconds. Repeat three times.

To perform eversion stretching, grip the left foot with the right hand—this time thumb near the bases of the toes and four fingers on the sole—and turn the sole outward (Fig. 36). It should take ten seconds and should be repeated three times.

Finally, supporting the left ankle with the left hand and gripping the toes of the left foot in the right hand, perform inward rotational stretching ten times and then outward rotational stretching ten times (one second each; Fig. 37).

Lateral Area of the Leg and the Sole of the Foot

● *Shiatsu*
Sitting either on the floor or in a chair, bend the left knee slightly inward and toward the left foot. Put the toes of the left foot on the floor in a stable position. The ten points for shiatsu on the lateral surface of the leg begin immediately below the head of the fibula and continue to the lateral malleolus (Fig. 38). Apply pressure to each for three seconds. Next put the left knee on the floor and turn the sole of the left foot upward. With the right thumb, apply pressure for three seconds to each of the five points beginning in the fleshy area below the base of the big toe and continuing on a diagonal line toward the heel (Fig. 38). Repeat these pressure applications on the lateral surface of the lower leg and on the sole of the foot three times.

The peroneus longus and peroneus brevis muscles, which cause eversion of the sole, are found in the region of the lateral surface of the leg and the sole of the foot. Stiffness in these muscles causes the body weight to shift to the outer part of the sole and thus upsets physical balance and brings on fatigue. Extreme wearing down of the outer sides of the heels of shoes, slipping when in a hurry, or a tendency to fall are symptoms of this condition. When they are observed, it is wise to perform shiatsu on the lateral surface of the leg and in this way to balance the weight load on the soles and stabilize foot movement. Though this shiatsu is a little difficult to perform on yourself, you should persevere because ignoring the symptoms mentioned above causes stiffness in the peroneus muscles.

● *Stretching*
Stand straight in front of a wall. Put your left hand on the wall for balance. Bend your left knee and bring the heel of the left foot to the buttocks, turning the toes of the left foot directly to the side and the sole up. Grip the foot firmly; the thumb of the right hand is on the sole, and the four fingers are wrapped around to the dorsal surface (Fig. 39). Next perform eversion stretching by rotating the sole of the foot outward and stretching the lower leg outward in the direction in which the toes of the

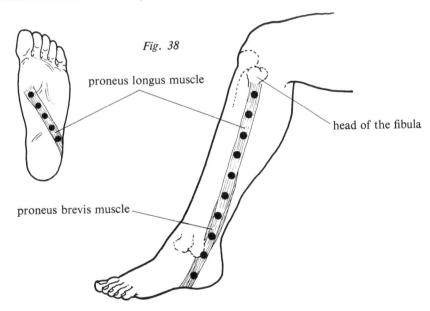

Fig. 38

proneus longus muscle

head of the fibula

proneus brevis muscle

left foot are pointed. Each stretch should last fifteen seconds; repeat three times. Next, in a similar fashion, while rotating the sole of the foot inward, perform inversion stretching by extending the lower leg inward in the direction in which the toes of the left foot point.

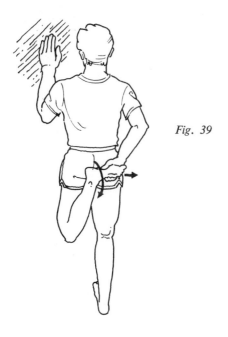

Fig. 39

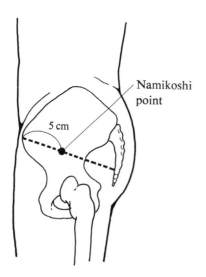

Fig. 40

Namikoshi point

5 cm

Effects of Treatment of the Anterior and Lateral Surfaces of the Lower Legs
Helpful in dealing with ambulatory insufficiency, chilling of the feet, contraction of the quadriceps femoris muscle, arthritis of the knee, hemiplegia, infantile paralysis, beriberi, treatment following a bone fracture, irregularities of the hip joint, rheumatism, swollen feet, knock-knees, bowlegs, talipes valgus, talipes varus, talipes equinus, and talipes calcaneus.

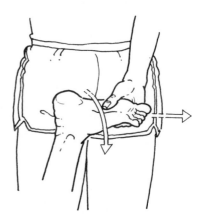

Namikoshi Points

● *Shiatsu*
Because they are distinctive to Namikoshi shiatsu, these points have been given this name. There are two of them, one on each side of the body five centimeters from the anterior superior iliac spine on a line connecting that spine and the sacrum (Fig. 40). Shiatsu pressure is applied to each Namikoshi point with the thumb, directed inward. The four fingers of each hand are wrapped around to the front of the body for support and are placed immediately below the anterior superior iliac spine. Begin with the left side and press deeply, with a gouging effect, to the side in the direction of the sacrum (Fig. 41). Press for five seconds. Repeat on the right side. Press three times on left and right sides in alternation.

Since the Namikoshi point is located on the gluteus medius muscle, pressure on it affects the sciatic nerve through the superior gluteal nerve and causes sharp pain. Stimulus caused by such pressure extends to the posterior side of the thigh, the anterior and posterior sides of the lower leg, and the toes. This in turn stimulates the functioning of the sciatic nerve, which is one of the thickest and longest of the peripheral nerves.

Effects
Treatment of this point helps cure the following conditions: sciatica, constipation, diarrhea, chilling of the feet, nocturnal enuresis, menstrual pains, stiff back, lumbago, urinary obstruction, fatigue in the lower limbs, rheumatism, beriberi, cramps, numbness of the legs, impotence, and frigidity.

Posterior Surface of the Thigh

• *Shiatsu*
This shiatsu is performed either in a position

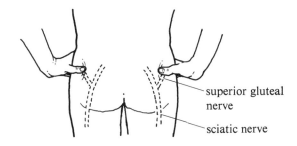

Fig. 41

superior gluteal nerve

sciatic nerve

seated on the floor with the legs outstretched and with the left (later the right) knee slightly bent or in a standing position with the left (later right) foot resting on a stool or low table. On the posterior surface of the thigh are three rows of ten points each leading from the gluteal fold to the popliteal fossa (Fig. 42). With the thumbs brought to the anterior surface of the thigh for support, press each of the points in the central row with the index, middle, and fourth

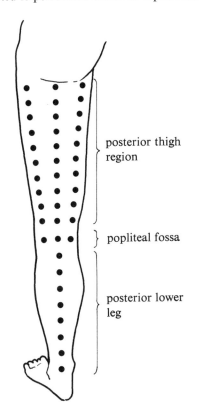

Fig. 42

posterior thigh region

popliteal fossa

posterior lower leg

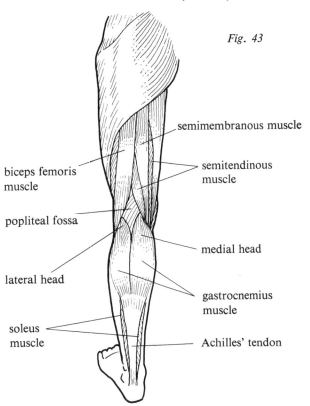

Fig. 43

semimembranous muscle

biceps femoris muscle

semitendinous muscle

popliteal fossa

medial head

lateral head

gastrocnemius muscle

soleus muscle

Achilles' tendon

fingers of the left and right hands—tips touching (Fig. 44). Each application should last for three seconds. Repeat three times. The sciatic nerve runs through this region. On both sides of it are the powerful muscles of the flexor group (called the hamstrings), which extend to the popliteal fossa (Fig. 43). This group of muscles actually creates this fossa and bends the knee, bringing the lower leg rearward to the posterior surface of the thigh and raising the foot to the buttocks. The tendons of the hamstrings can be felt on either side of the popliteal fossa: on the lateral side the tendon of the biceps femoris muscle and on the medial side the tendons of the semitendinous and semimembranous muscles.

Next, with the index, middle, and fourth fingers of the right and left hands, simultane-. ously press the lateral and medial rows of points beginning immediately below the gluteal

fold and continuing to the popliteal fossa (Fig. 42). Each application should last three seconds; repeat three times.

Popliteal Fossa

● *Shiatsu*

Simultaneously, with the index, middle, and fourth fingers of right and left hands, press the tendons on either side of the fossa. Then, in the same way, tips touching, press the central part (Fig. 45). Each pressure application should last three seconds. Repeat three times. Limbering the popliteal fossa by means of shiatsu strengthens the knees and facilitates their functioning.

● *Stretching*

With your back to a wall, press your buttocks against the wall surface, extend both legs forward, press both heels against the floor, and slightly raise your toes. When you are balanced in this position, incline your trunk slightly forward and, holding your arms straight, grip both thighs above the knees with both hands and push downward (Fig. 46). Hold this position for ten seconds and repeat three times. The important thing is to maintain balance with the three points of contact: buttocks, knees, and heels and to keep the back, arms, and legs straight.

Fig. 44

Fig. 45

Fig. 46

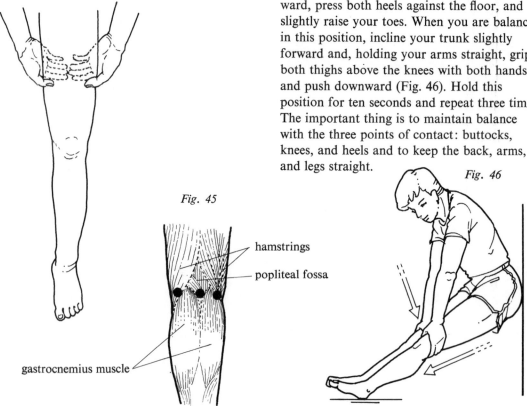

hamstrings

popliteal fossa

gastrocnemius muscle

Next, standing straight, put the heel of the left foot on a stool or low table. Keep the left leg straight and the body stable. Stretch the posterior side of the thigh and the popliteal fossa by placing the palms of the right and left hands on the thigh just in front of the knee and pressing straight down (Fig. 47). Hold for ten seconds and repeat three times.

Posterior Side of the Lower Leg (Calf)

● *Shiatsu*
Sitting on the floor with legs outstretched forward or sitting in a chair, bend the left knee and open it outward. Place the left ankle lightly on the right foot and thus turn the left calf toward your body. Three muscles are responsible for the bulge called the calf: the medial and lateral heads of the gastrocnemius muscle and the soleus muscle; collectively, they are known as the triceps femoris. They connect with the heel by means of the Achilles' tendon (see Fig. 43). The triceps femoris is responsible for plantarflexion of the foot and for such motions as rising on the toes.

To perform shiatsu on this region, place the left hand on the left knee. With the fingers ex-

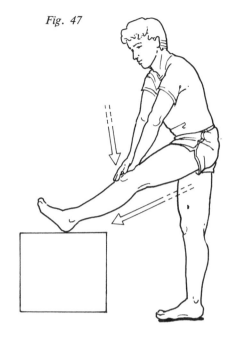

Fig. 47

tended forward for support, press with the tip of the right thumb (turned upward) on each of the eight points aligned down the center of the calf from the popliteal fossa to immediately in front of the Achilles' tendon (Figs. 42 and 48). Press for three seconds and repeat three times.

The next procedure is to squeeze the entire calf by pressing the right thumb against the

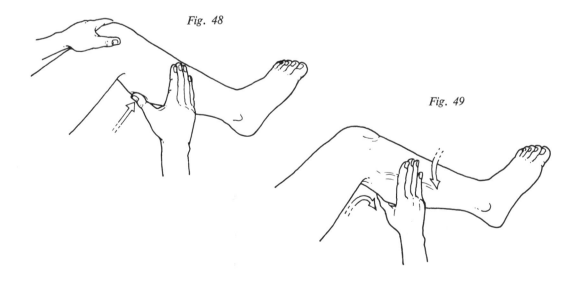

Fig. 48

Fig. 49

Fig. 50

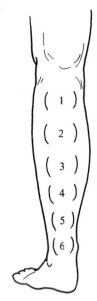

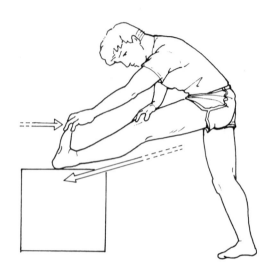

Fig. 51

lateral gastrocnemius muscle and the four fingers of the right hand against the medial gastrocnemius muscle and squeezing them upward (Fig. 49). The thumb and fingers should bend inward to lift the muscles directly upward. Beginning at the one immediately below the popliteal fossa, squeeze in this manner at each of the six points on the calf (Fig. 50). Hold each squeeze three seconds then release. Repeat each three times.

● *Stretching*

Standing, put the heel of the left foot on a stool or low table. Keep the leg straight and turn the toes upward. Place the right hand on the left thigh, immediately in front of the knee. Dorsiflex the sole of the left foot by gripping all its toes in the left hand and pulling them forward (Fig. 51). Hold for ten seconds and repeat three times.

To stretch the calf, stand with both hands on a wall, with the right foot forward, with the left foot drawn back, and with both feet flat on the floor (Fig. 52). Leaving both feet on the floor, lightly bend the right knee and slowly lean the trunk forward. Hold for ten seconds and repeat three times.

Fig. 52

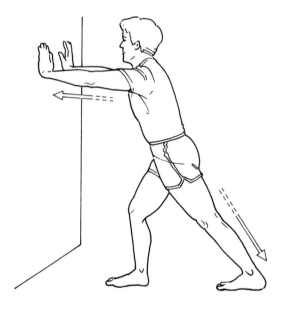

Heel

• *Shiatsu and Stretching*
In treating the heel, shiatsu and stretching are carried out simultaneously. Bend the left knee and put the left ankle on the right knee. Pull the left heel forward. Supporting the ankle with the left hand, with the tip of the right thumb (pointed toward the sole), bring the four fingers of the right hand to the lateral side of the ankle. Three shiatsu points are located between the heel and the Achilles' tendon. Press each with an upward kneading motion (Figs. 53 and 54). Each pressure application lasts three seconds; repeat three times.

Next, gripping the center of the Achilles' tendon slightly above the malleolus, stretch it alternately upward and downward rapidly and rhythmically ten times (Fig. 55).

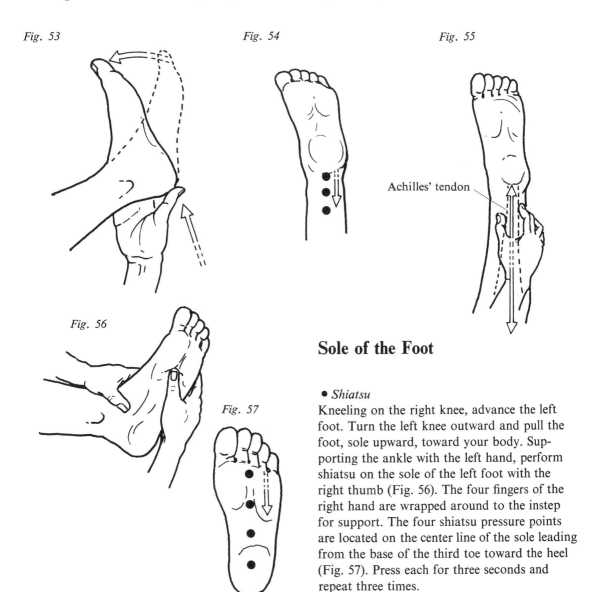

Fig. 53

Fig. 54

Fig. 55

Achilles' tendon

Fig. 56

Fig. 57

Sole of the Foot

• *Shiatsu*
Kneeling on the right knee, advance the left foot. Turn the left knee outward and pull the foot, sole upward, toward your body. Supporting the ankle with the left hand, perform shiatsu on the sole of the left foot with the right thumb (Fig. 56). The four fingers of the right hand are wrapped around to the instep for support. The four shiatsu pressure points are located on the center line of the sole leading from the base of the third toe toward the heel (Fig. 57). Press each for three seconds and repeat three times.

Fig. 58

A. cervical vertebrae
B. thoracic vertebrae
C. lumbar vertebrae

D. sacrum
E. coccyx

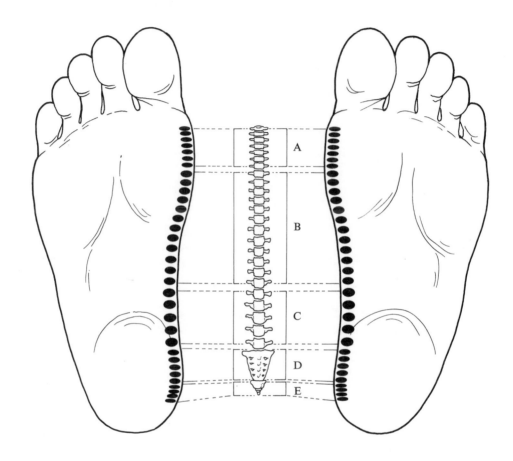

Fig. 59

Fig. 60

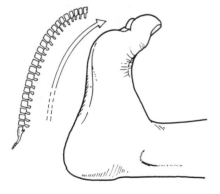

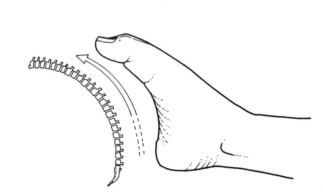

Walking on pavement and other hard, flat surfaces, as today we are often compelled to do for long times, causes the sole to lose its natural flexibility. Furthermore, because of the intimate connection between them, when the back grows stiff, so does the sole (Figs. 58–60). It is consequently necessary to keep the muscles of the sole limber; and thorough shiatsu on the inner side of the sole is especially vital.

● *Stretching*
In the same position as for shiatsu, put the left hand on the left ankle. The thumb of the right hand is on the dorsal surface of the left foot at the base of the toes, and the four fingers are brought around to the sole. Dorsiflex the foot by pushing the toes well forward (Fig. 61). Then plantarflex the left foot. Repeat dorsiflexion and plantarflexion, alternately, three times for ten seconds each time.

Near a wall place a brick, concrete block, or something similar on which you can stand and shift your weight without losing balance. Supporting yourself with both hands on the wall, stand on the brick with your toes projecting beyond the edge and, maintaining good balance, shift your weight to the front to cause dorsi-

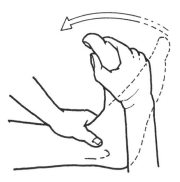

Fig. 61

flexion stretching (Fig. 62). Hold for ten seconds. Then stand on the brick so that your heels extend beyond the edge. Once again, maintaining good balance, shift your weight rearward to cause plantarflexion of the foot (Fig. 63). Repeat the two, alternately, three times each.

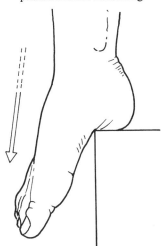

Fig. 62

plantarflexion stretching

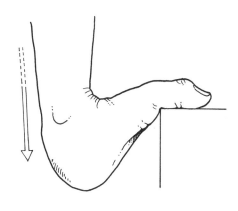

Fig. 63

dorsiflexion stretching

70

• *Shiatsu and Stretching with Both Feet*
This kind of shiatsu and stretching is done lying on the back on the floor and with the feet. First, lying on the floor, outstretch the left leg and open it outward. Bend the right leg and, with the right foot, apply shiatsu pressure to the six points on a line extending down the calf from the popliteal fossa to the ankle (Fig. 64). Each pressure application should last three seconds; repeat three times. Repeat pressure on the same six points but round the right foot inward as much as possible (Fig. 65). Each application lasts for three seconds; repeat three times. In the same position, rub with the sole of the right foot up and down the calf

rapidly ten times (Fig. 66).

Next shiatsu is performed on the sole of the foot. Bending both knees, with the big toe of the right foot, apply pressure to the four points on the center of the sole of the left foot from the bases of the toes to the heel (Fig. 67). Each application lasts three seconds; repeat three times. Then, with the heel of the right foot, apply strong pressure for five seconds to the arch of the left foot (Fig. 68). Repeat three times.

Dorsiflexion and plantarflexion are carried out for the sole of the foot. Dorsiflexion is performed lying on the back. With the left leg outstretched, pull the toes of the left foot

Fig. 64

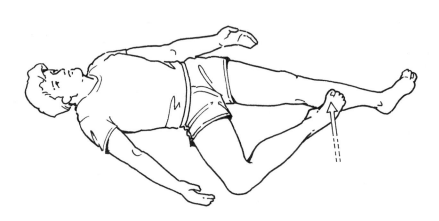

Fig. 65

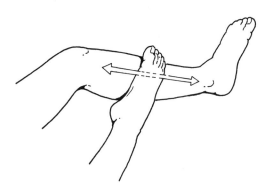

Fig. 66

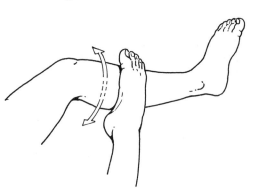

Fig. 67

Fig. 68

Fig. 69

Fig. 70

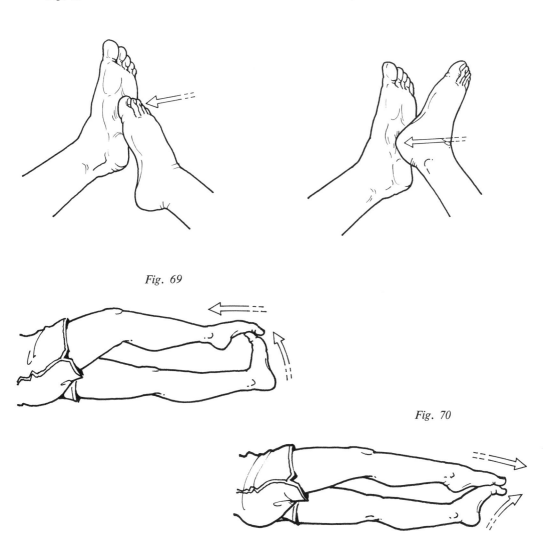

forward with the toes of the right foot (Fig. 69). Hold the stretch position ten seconds and repeat three times. Plantarflexion is performed in a similar manner, except that the toes of the right foot push the toes of the left foot outward (Fig. 70). Hold the stretch position ten seconds and repeat three times. Performed daily before going to sleep at night and before rising in the morning, this kind of two-leg shiatsu and stretching makes many daily bodily motions lighter and easier.

Effects of Treatment on the Posterior Regions of the Lower Limbs

This treatment brings relief from the following conditions: sciatica, cramps, rheumatism, knock-knees and bowlegs, partial knock-knees, arthritis of the knee, contraction of the Achilles' tendon, chilling in the legs, hemiplegia, infantile paralysis, irregularities in the hip joint, beriberi, sprains, talipes valgus, talipes varus, talipes calcaneus, and ambulatory insufficiencies. In addition, it is good therapy after a bone fracture.

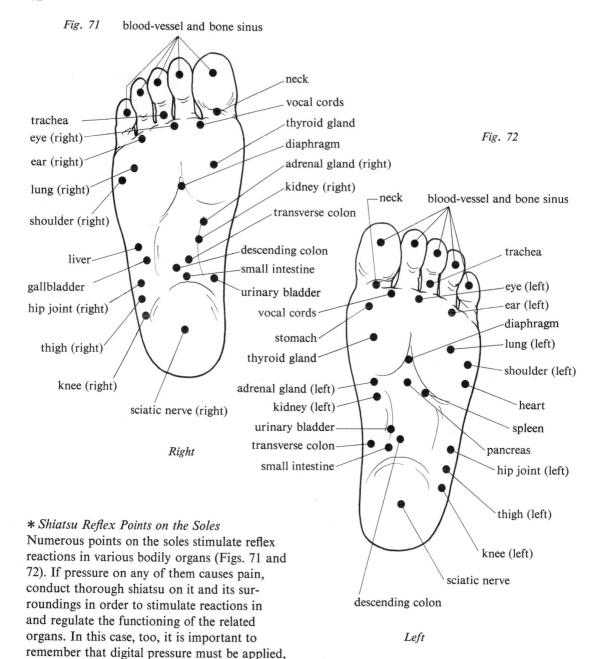

Fig. 71   blood-vessel and bone sinus

neck
vocal cords
thyroid gland
trachea
eye (right)
diaphragm
ear (right)
adrenal gland (right)
lung (right)
kidney (right)
shoulder (right)
transverse colon

Fig. 72

descending colon
liver
small intestine
gallbladder
urinary bladder
hip joint (right)

thigh (right)

knee (right)

sciatic nerve (right)

Right

neck   blood-vessel and bone sinus

trachea
eye (left)
ear (left)
diaphragm
lung (left)
shoulder (left)

heart
spleen
pancreas
hip joint (left)

vocal cords
stomach
thyroid gland
adrenal gland (left)
kidney (left)
urinary bladder
transverse colon
small intestine

thigh (left)

knee (left)

sciatic nerve

descending colon

Left

∗ Shiatsu Reflex Points on the Soles
Numerous points on the soles stimulate reflex
reactions in various bodily organs (Figs. 71 and
72). If pressure on any of them causes pain,
conduct thorough shiatsu on it and its sur-
roundings in order to stimulate reactions in
and regulate the functioning of the related
organs. In this case, too, it is important to
remember that digital pressure must be applied,
not recklessly and with too much force, but
gradually and gently so that it penetrates
pleasantly. In other words, shiatsu is effective
only when the right amount of pressure is applied to the right place.

Even people who get plenty of daily exercise
through sports tend to overlook care of the
feet. Shiatsu on the soles, which can be performed easily even by the elderly, improves
circulation without putting a burden on the
heart. Taking the time to execute this and
shiatsu for the lower limbs in general has a
rejuvenating effect.

5. Shiatsu and Stretching for the Back

In this connection, the word *back* refers to the spinal column and its thirty-three vertebrae: seven cervical vertebrae, twelve thoracic vertebrae, five lumbar vertebrae, five sacral vertebrae, and the four rudimentary vertebrae of the coccyx. These vertebrae play the important role of supporting the head and maintaining erect posture. The twenty-three cartilaginous intervertebral discs act as shock absorbers for the vertebrae. Numerous erector spinae muscles make possible anterior, posterior, left, and right twisting and bending of the spinal column. Insufficient exercise or fatigue hardens these muscles, thus inhibiting the flow of nutrients to the vertebrae and intervertebral discs through the blood and lymph. As a consequence, the back is deformed; and the intervertebral discs shrink to the point where they can easily slip out of proper position. It is important to prevent this by getting sufficient daily exercise and performing the shiatsu and stretching outlined below to limber the muscles of the back.

Fig. 1

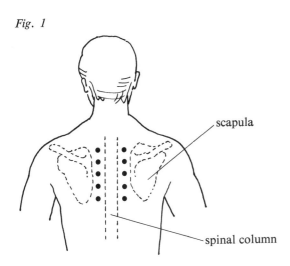
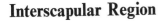

scapula

spinal column

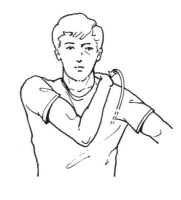

Fig. 2

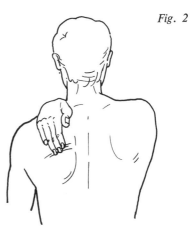

Interscapular Region

● *Shiatsu*
Shiatsu for the back begins with the interscapular region (Fig. 1). Because this is the part of the body most inaccessible to one's own hands, self-shiatsu for it requires special operational techniques.

There are two rows of five shiatsu points on either side of the back between the spinal column and the scapulae. To perform shiatsu

Fig. 3

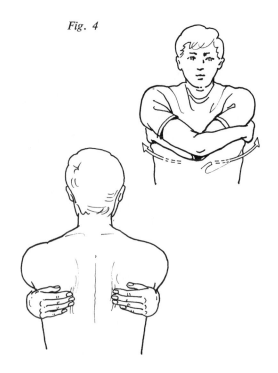

Fig. 4

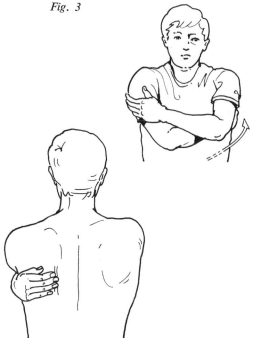

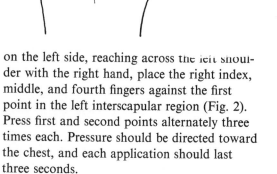

on the left side, reaching across the left shoulder with the right hand, place the right index, middle, and fourth fingers against the first point in the left interscapular region (Fig. 2). Press first and second points alternately three times each. Pressure should be directed toward the chest, and each application should last three seconds.

Next, extend the left arm forward, bend the elbow, and relax the arm. Passing the right hand under the left arm, with the right index, middle, and fourth fingers, press the third shiatsu point in the left interscapular region (Fig. 3). Press this point and points four and five for three seconds each. Repeat three times. The pressure should be directed toward the chest.

When treatment on the left side has been completed, perform the same kind of treatment on the right side.

Finally, shiatsu is applied to both sides simultaneously. Crossing the arms in front of the chest, press the inner boundary of the first point in the left interscapular region with the index, middle, and fourth fingers of the right

hand and the inner boundary of the first point in the right interscapular region with the index, middle, and fourth fingers of the left hand (Fig. 4). The pressure should be applied in an outward pulling fashion. Each application should last three seconds. Repeat three times. Continue to press in the same way all of the remaining points on both sides. This shiatsu has the simultaneous effect of opening the scapulae outward and thus stretching the muscles of the interscapular region. When you have become able to perform this treatment easily, you will have mastered a highly sophisticated shiatsu and stretching technique.

Infrascapular and Lumber Regions

● *Shiatsu and Stretching*
Below the interscapular region are two rows of five points each in the infrascapular region and two rows of five each below these in the lumbar region, extending from the fifth lumbar vertebra to the sacrum (Fig. 5). Shiatsu is applied to the

Fig. 5

Fig. 6

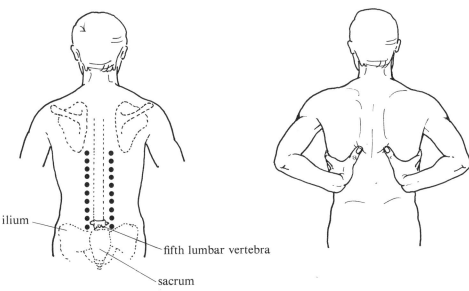

ilium

fifth lumbar vertebra

sacrum

left and right rows simultaneously with the thumbs, turned up (Fig. 6). The four fingers of each hand are wrapped around toward the abdomen. Pressure is directed toward the abdomen. Each application lasts three seconds. Repeat each three times. Ideally, in pressing the first infrascapular points, place your thumbs as close to the bottom edges of the scapulae as possible; that is, the thumbs should be immediately below the scapulae.

Stretching consists in simultaneously pushing upward and pulling downward with the thumbs on each point in the left and right rows with short movements (Fig. 7). Each push should last three seconds. Execute one full series of these stretching motions. In this region are

Fig. 7

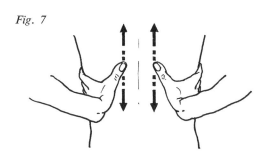

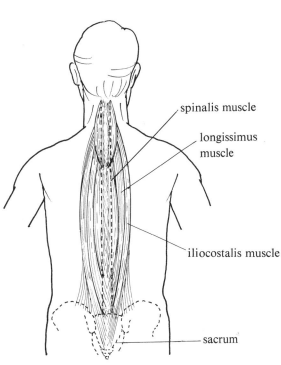

spinalis muscle

longissimus muscle

iliocostalis muscle

sacrum

erector spinae muscle

Fig. 8

located bundles of muscles collectively called the erector spinae muscles—spinalis and longissimus adjacent to the spinal column and iliocostalis on the outer side—that control the motion of the spinal column (Fig. 8). Stretching in this area limbers the erector spinae muscles and makes its motion smooth. Effectiveness is further increased, if the exercise is performed in the bath or lying on the side in bed, when the muscles are relaxed. In such a position, beginning on the left side, with the index, middle, and fourth fingers, press the five interscapular points and the ten in the infrascapular and lumbar regions (Fig. 9).

Sacral Region

• *Shiatsu*
The erector spinae muscles, which arise in the sacral region, extend from the iliac crest to the lumbar vertebrae, the ribs, the thoracic vertebrae, and the cervical vertebrae. There are three shiatsu points on the sacrum (Fig. 10). Pressure is applied to them, with the tips of both thumbs touching, pointed up, and with the four fingers of each hand turned straight to the side (Fig. 11). Each pressure application lasts three seconds. Repeat three times. Since the points are located directly on the sacrum, pressure must be gentle and moderate.

• *Stretching the Back*
Lie supine on the floor with a cushion under your back. First extend your arms above your

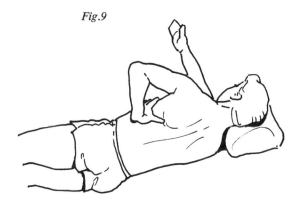
Fig.9

head and relax. Then stretch your back by vigorously extending arms upward and legs downward (Fig. 12). After holding the extended position for ten seconds, return to the original relaxed position. Repeat three times.

Next, still lying on your back, remove the cushion. Interlock the fingers of both hands and, with the palms turned upward, extend both arms above your head. Without moving the lower part of your body, bend your trunk, head, and arms as far as possible to the left (Fig. 13). Hold this stretched position for ten seconds. Return to the starting position. Repeat three times then execute the same stretching exercise to the right three times.

Sitting in a chair, interlock the fingers of both hands. Pressing the thenars of both hands close against the occipital bone, bend your trunk as far forward as possible (Fig. 14). Hold the stretched position ten seconds. Return to the starting position. Repeat three times.

Fig. 10

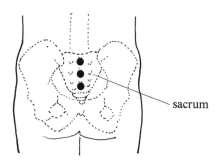
sacrum

Fig. 11

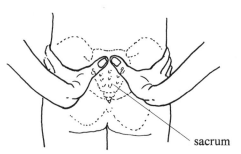
sacrum

Fig. 12

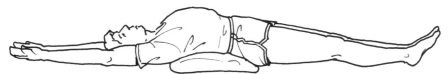

Fig. 13

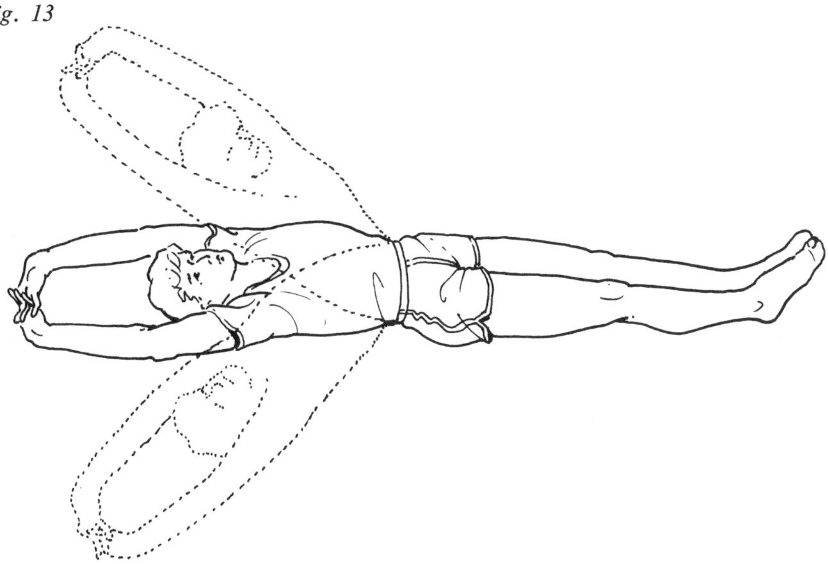

Fig. 14

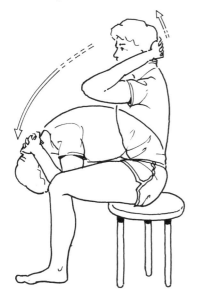

Lying on your back, wrap your arms around your legs just below the knees. Pull you knees to your body. Reduce the distance between them further by raising your head off the floor (Fig. 15). Hold this stretched position ten seconds. Return head and legs to the floor and relax. Repeat three times.

Fig. 15

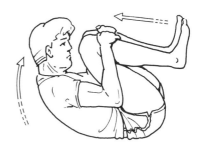

Next contract the back by lying prone, bending the knees, and bringing both feet—held together—close to the upper body. Hold them with both hands by the instep near the toes. Further raise both the legs and the trunk (Fig. 16). Hold this stretched position ten seconds. Release the hold you have with your hands and, leaving your knees bent, relax, lowering your trunk to the floor. Repeat three times.

Standing straight with legs spread slightly apart. Raise both arms above your head. Bend your left elbow and let your left forearm rest on your head. Bend your right elbow and let your right forearm lie along your left one. Stretch the back by bending your trunk as far left as possible (Fig. 17). Hold the stretched position for ten seconds. Return to the upright position. Repeat three times. Perform the same stretching exercise to the right side.

For the twisting exercise, stand straight with legs slightly spread apart (Fig. 18). Position a chair, with a back, conveniently close to and

Fig. 16

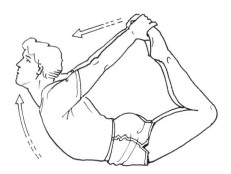

behind you. Without moving your legs or feet, twist your trunk as far as possible to the left. Grip the back of the chair, and hold this position for ten seconds (Fig. 19). Repeat three times. Perform stretching exercises to the right in the same fashion.

Fig. 17   *Fig. 18*   *Fig. 19*

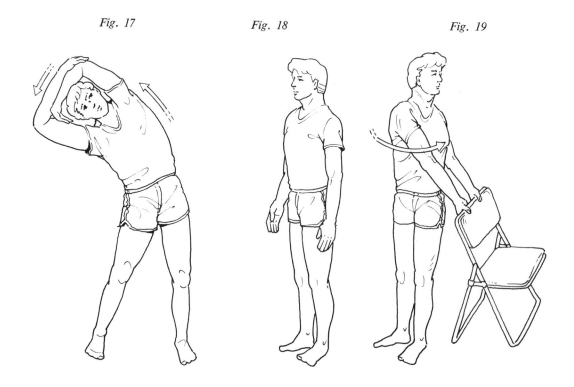

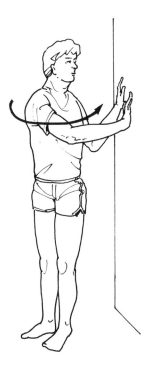

Fig. 20

Another twisting exercise is performed using a wall for support. Standing straight with legs slightly spread apart, about thirty centimeters in front of a wall, turn your trunk as far as possible to the left. Bring both arms to the rear, lightly bend your elbows, and place both hands on the wall higher than shoulder height (Fig. 20). Hold this stretched position for ten seconds. Return your trunk to the starting position. Repeat three times. Then perform the same twist to the right three times.

Next stand, feet together, facing a wall, about fifty centimeters from it. Raise both arms and hold them about shoulders' width apart. Place both palms on the wall. Without altering the positions of hands or feet and keeping both soles flat on the floor, bend your knees and lower your body forward slightly (Figs. 21 and 22). Hold the stretched position for twenty seconds then return to the starting position. Repeat three times.

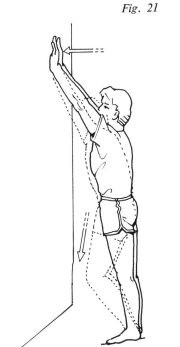

Fig. 21

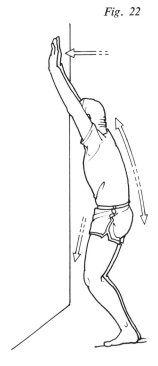

Fig. 22

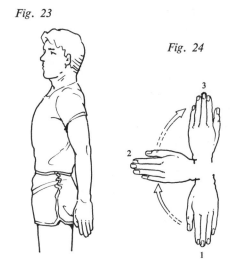

Fig. 23

Fig. 24

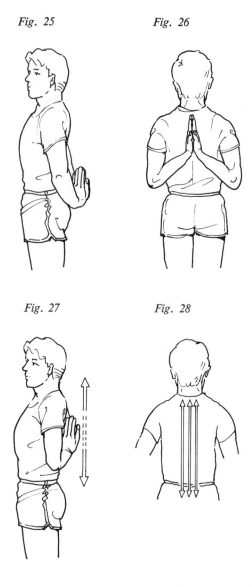

Fig. 25

Fig. 26

Fig. 27

Fig. 28

● *Palmar and Digital Stimulation of the Spinal Nerve*

Stimulating the reflexes of the spinal nerve improves its functioning and orders the functioning of all the internal organs related to it. At the same time, this treatment limbers the muscle groups on both sides of the spinal column. Since it is performed with the hands held behind the back, this therapy demands flexibility in the muscles of the arms and smooth movement of the shoulder and elbow joints. Consequently, it must be performed only after a thorough warm-up of the arms.

Standing in a comfortable position, bring both arms behind you and, fingers pointed down, join your palms (Fig. 23). Turn your hands so that the fingers point toward your body. Continue turning them until your fingers point up and your little fingers lie along your spinal column (Figs. 24 and 25).

Next, slide your hands as far upward as possible, leaving your little fingers pressed against your spinal column (Fig. 26). This is the position from which palmar-digital stimulation of the spinal nerve begins. With the little fingers constantly in contact with the spinal column, lower both hands, stroking the back downward (Fig. 27). Then, raising them to the maximum height, stroke it upward. The raising and lowering must be quick. Repeat the full cycle ten times.

Then, sliding the little fingers first to the left and then to the right of the spinal column, repeat the same raising and lowering ten times on each side (Fig. 28).

Effects of Treatment on the Back

Regulation of the functioning of the internal organs, limbering the erector spinae muscles; regulation of the intervertebral discs; and prevention of ossification of the vertebral ligaments, kyphosis, lordosis, scoliosis, flat back, lumbago, sciatica, and vertebral deformation.

6.   Shiatsu and Stretching for the Head

To perform this treatment, cover the head with a thin towel or piece of cotton cloth to prevent pulling the hair and soiling the fingers with hair oils and other cosmetics. The cloth may be dispensed with if the treatment is performed immediately after washing the hair.

● *Shiatsu on the Parietal Median Line*
Six shiatsu points are aligned along the parietal median line from the hairline. Apply pressure to each with the overlapped index, middle, and fourth fingers of both hands, right hand on the

bottom. Each application should last for three seconds. The pressure should be perpendicular to the surface of the head (Figs. 1 and 2). Repeat three times.

● *Shiatsu on the Temporal Region*
On either side of each of the six points on the median line are rows of six points leading across the temporal region to the lateral and rear hairlines (Fig. 3). With the index, middle, and fourth fingers of each hand, press each point in the rows leading left and right from the

Fig. 1

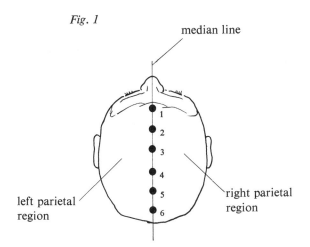

median line

left parietal region

right parietal region

Fig. 2

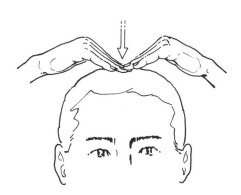

Fig. 3

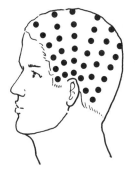

Fig. 4

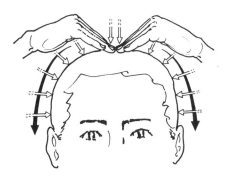

Fig. 5

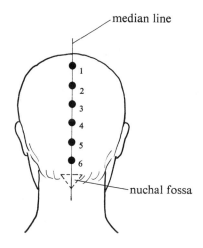

median line

1
2
3
4
5
6

nuchal fossa

Fig. 7

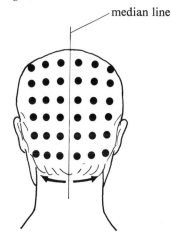

median line

Fig. 8

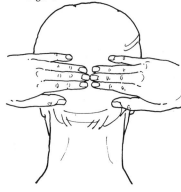

Fig. 6

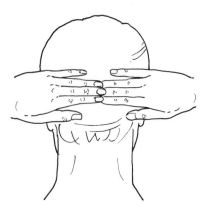

sixth point on the median line (Fig. 4). In the same fashion, continue with the lines of points starting with the fifth, fourth, and so on until you have completed all of the lines, ending with the ones leading left and right from the first point on the median line. Each pressure application should last three seconds and should be perpendicular to the surface of the head.

● *Shiatsu on the Occipital Region*
The median line of six points for the occipital region begins immediately behind the sixth point in the parietal median line and continues to the medulla oblongata (nuchal fossa). With the overlapped index, middle, and fourth fingers of both hands (right hand on the bottom) press each of these points for three seconds (Figs. 5 and 6). Repeat three times.

Beside those on the occipital median line on each side of the head are six rows of three points each, extending to the hairline (Fig. 7). With the index, middle, and fourth fingers of each hand, simultaneously press each point leading left and right from the sixth point on the median line, then the fifth, fourth, and so on till all six pairs have been treated (Fig. 8). Each application of pressure lasts three seconds. Repeat three times.

● *Stretching the Head*
Though it seems to be all in one piece, the skull is actually composed of a combination of several bones. For instance, in the region enclosing

Fig. 9

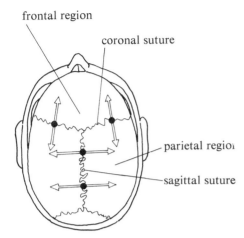

frontal region

coronal suture

parietal region

sagittal suture

Fig. 10

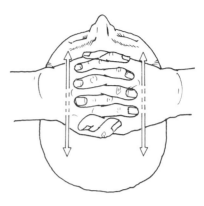

Fig. 11

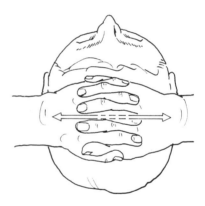

Fig. 12

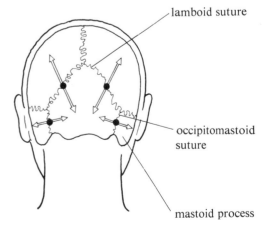

lamboid suture

occipitomastoid suture

mastoid process

the brain alone there are seven, all connected by sutures. These sutures gradually close with increasing age and brain development until, ultimately, the cranial bones fuse. Though it differs with the individual, the process of fusion of the cranial bones is slower than that of any other bones in the human body. Shiatsu pressure and stretching applied to these sutures stimulate and activate the functioning of the brain.

First, perform stretching of the coronal suture (Fig. 9), which does not completely close until the age of about forty. Stretch it by interlocking the fingers of both hands, which are then put on top of the head. Move the hands forward one second and rearward one second (Fig. 10). Repeat three times.

To stretch the sagittal suture, which closes completely at the age of about thirty-five (Fig. 9), interlock the hands as in the preceding stretching exercise, and move the palms of the hands right for one second then left for one second (Fig. 11). Repeat three times.

In the occipital region of the head is the lamboid suture (Fig. 12), which closes completely at about the age of forty-five. Stretch it by interlocking the fingers of both hands and pressing the palms against the occipital region. Then, in a pattern that widens at the top, move the palms diagonally upward for one second

Fig. 13

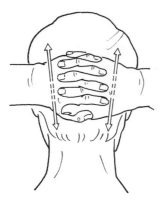

Fig. 14

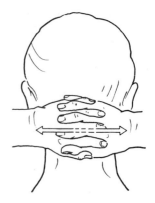

then downward for one second. Repeat three times (Fig. 13).

Below the occipital bone is the occipito-mastoid suture (Fig. 12), which does not completely close until the age of about eighty. With the fingers of both hands interlocked, press the palms against the area to the sides of the mastoid process and pull them one second to the right and one second to the left (Fig. 14). Repeat three times.

The zygomaticofrontal suture, located in the temporal region (Fig. 15), does not completely close until the age of about sixty-five. Stretch it by placing the digital balls of the index, middle, and fourth fingers of each hand (fingers pointed upward) on the area slightly above the outer ends of the eyes. Simultaneously raise and lower the fingers on both sides for one second each (Fig. 16).

Fig. 15

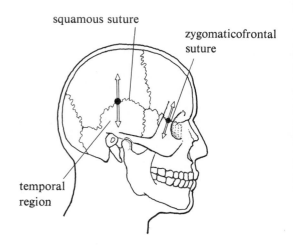

squamous suture

zygomaticofrontal suture

temporal region

Fig. 16

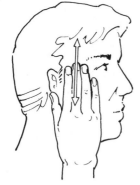

Fig. 17

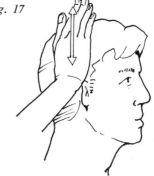

The squamous suture, in the temporal region (Fig. 15), does not close until the age of about eighty. With the fingers together and pointed upward, press the palms against the temporal regions on both sides of the head simultaneously. Move the hands upward for one second then downward for one second (Fig. 17). Repeat three times.

When these shiatsu and stretching treatments have been completed, further stimulate the brain by means of light vibration treatment to all regions of the head (Fig. 18).

Fig. 18

vibration technique

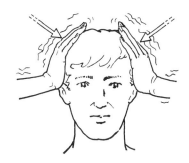

Fig. 19

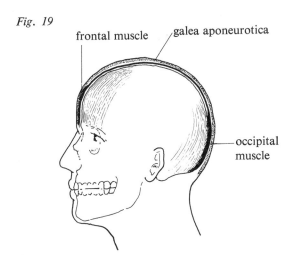

frontal muscle

galea aponeurotica

occipital muscle

Fig. 20

auricular muscles

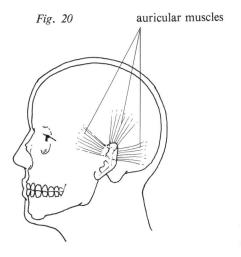

● *Stretching the Hair*

Proper care can prevent the premature graying and balding that are increasingly prevalent among young people today. Unless steps are taken, subcutaneous fat accumulates under the scalp, weakening metabolism, making the scalp go slack, and thus causing hair to fall out or turn gray (see Figs. 19–21). At the same time, the skin of the face becomes wrinkled and flaccid. Care of the face alone will not solve the problem since it is necessary to treat the scalp first. When the scalp is in good condition, the skin of the face will regain its smoothness, luster, and youthfulness. Extremely effective in this connection, the hair-stretching regimen outlined below stimulates the scalp and hair roots, thus improving circulation and nourishment of

Fig. 21

temporal muscle

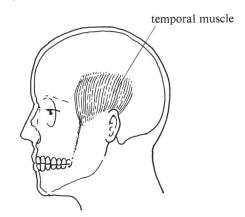

Fig. 22

Fig. 23

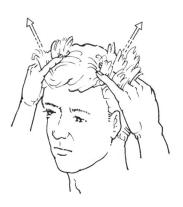

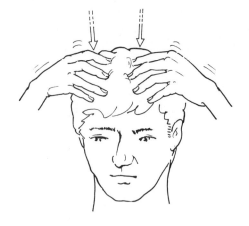

Fig. 24

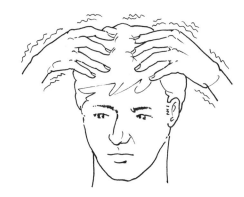

the hair. Without resorting to daily artificial treatments, with this shiatsu and stretching routine, you can keep your hair naturally lustrous.

After washing and thoroughly drying the hair, first perform the shiatsu for the head described in the preceding pages. Then, with the five fingers of each hand, grip the hair near the roots and pull it (Fig. 22). Moving the hands from place to place all over the head, continue pulling rhythmically, one second per place, for from two to three minutes.

Next, spreading the fingers slightly, apply the digital balls to the scalp. The fingers should be raised slightly. Moving the fingers from place to place, apply shiatsu pressure rhythmically for from two to three minutes, one second an application over the entire scalp (Fig. 23). Then, with the digital balls of the five fingers of both hands, vibrate the whole scalp (Fig. 24). Each vibration should last five seconds.

Effects

This treatment helps prevent insomnia, headaches, migraine, heaviness of the head, undernourished hair, failing memory, neuroses, premature senility, senile dementia, alopecia areata, and occipital neuralgia.

7. Shiatsu and Stretching for the Face

● *Shiatsu on the Forehead*
Between the glabella and hairline on the median line of the face are three shiatsu points (Fig. 1). With the overlapped index, middle, and fourth fingers of both hands (right hand on the bottom), press each of these points from the lowest to the highest for three seconds each (Fig. 2). Repeat three times. On either side of the second of the three points on the median line is a horizontal line of three points. With the index, middle, and fourth fingers of both hands, simultaneously press each point for three seconds, from the inner side outward. Repeat three times (Fig. 3).

Fig. 1

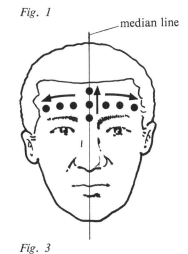

median line

Fig. 2

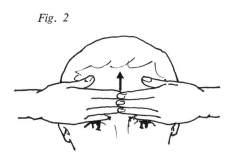

Fig. 3

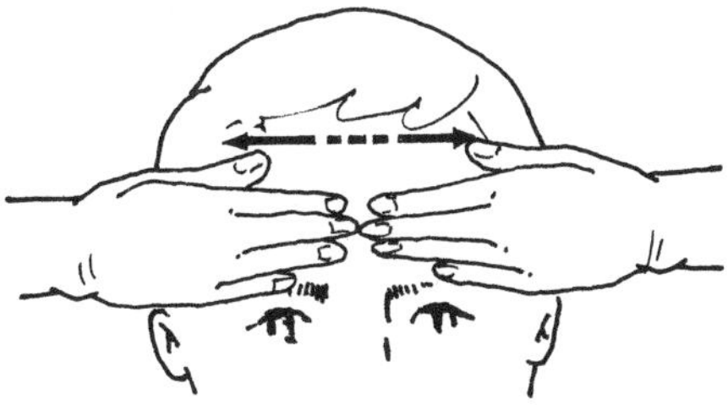

Fig. 4

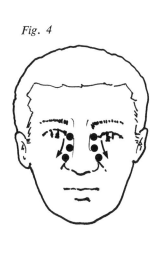

Fig. 5

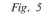

● *Shiatsu on Either Side of the Nose*
On each side of the nose, beginning at the inner edges of the eyes and extending to the nostrils, is a row of three shiatsu points (Fig. 4). Simultaneously, with the middle finger resting on its nail, press each point with the digital ball of the index finger for three seconds (Fig. 5). Repeat three times.

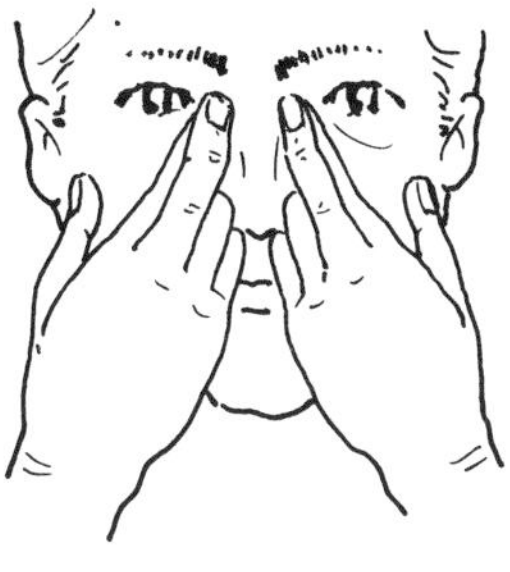

Fig. 6

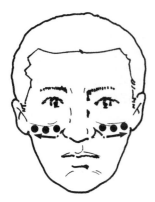

Fig. 7

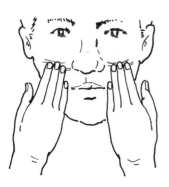

Fig. 10

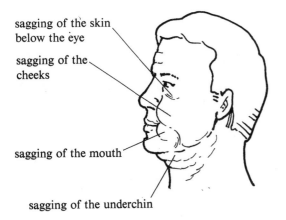

sagging of the skin
below the eye

sagging of the
cheeks

sagging of the mouth

sagging of the underchin

• *Shiatsu on the Zygomatic Region*

Align the index, middle, and fourth fingers of
each hand on the inner edge of the zygomatic
bone (Figs. 6 and 7). Beginning at the first
point, adjacent to the nose, press each of the
points in the two horizontal lines lying along
the zygomatic bone. Pressure should be applied
in a forward pulling fashion. Each application
should last three seconds. Repeat three times.
This shiatsu effectively tightens the skin of the
cheeks (see Fig. 10).

Fig. 8

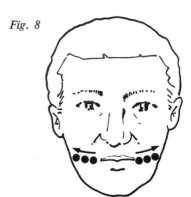

Fig. 9

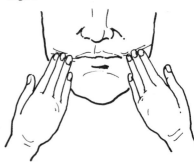

• *Shiatsu for the Mouth*

Using the same fingers as in shiatsu for the
zygomatic region, apply pressure to each of the
two rows of three points leading from each
corner of the mouth to the mandibular angle
(Figs. 8 and 9). Each application should last
three seconds. Repeat three times. This shiatsu
effectively corrects sagging of the mouth (see
Fig. 10).

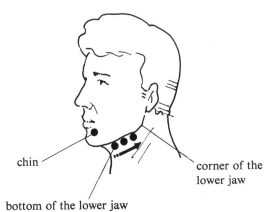

Fig. 11

chin

bottom of the lower jaw

corner of the
lower jaw

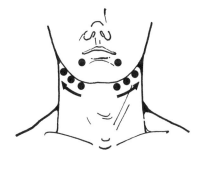

Fig. 12

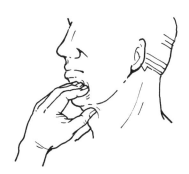

Fig. 13

● *Shiatsu for the Mandible*
With the index, middle, and fourth fingers of
each hand placed together in the mental foramen below the outer tips of the mouth, press
simultaneously with the thumbs the two rows of
three points along the under edge of the mandibular bone, beginning just below the mental
foramen and continuing to the mandibular
angle (Figs. 11–13). This shiatsu prevents sagging of the underchin (see Fig. 10) and stimulates the secretion of the salivary glands.

● *Shiatsu for the Region around the Eyes*
A supraorbital and an infraorbital row of four
points each surround each eye (Fig. 14). In
applying shiatsu to them, care must be taken
not to press directly on the eye itself. Beginning
with the innermost points in the infraorbital

fossa, apply pressure simultaneously to the left
and right rows with the index, middle, and
fourth fingers of each hand. Each application
should last for three seconds. Repeat three
times, then execute the same kind of treatment
on the supraorbital fossae (Fig. 15).

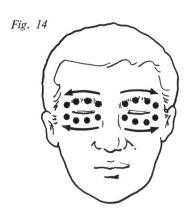

Fig. 14

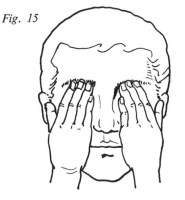

Fig. 15

Next, using the same fingers, apply pressure to each point in the three rows extending from the outermost tip of each eye across the temporal region (Figs. 16 and 17). Pressure should be applied as if it were a pull in the direction of the ear. Press each point three seconds and repeat three times.

Fig. 16

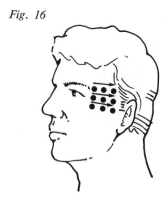

• *Stretching the Forehead*
Place the index, middle, and fourth fingers of each hand—held horizontally—on each side of the forehead median line above the glabella. Pressing the digital balls tightly against the skin, simultaneously slide the fingers upward on both right and left sides, stopping at the hairline (Fig. 18). Hold for ten seconds. Release the fingers and relax. Repeat three times.

For horizontal stretching of the forehead, place the index, middle, and fourth fingers of each hand beside the forehead median line. Then, with a pulling motion, slide the fingers straight to the right and left sides simultaneously as far as the temporal hair line (Fig. 19). Perform this stretching for ten seconds then release the fingers and relax. Repeat three times.

Fig. 17

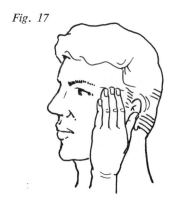

Fig. 18

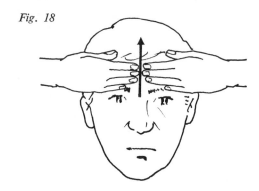

Fig. 19

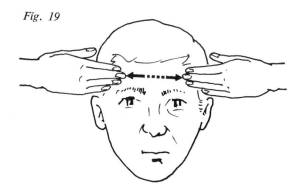

• *Stretching the Nostrils*
First limber the muscles in the region by performing shiatsu on both sides of the nose. Then, with the left index finger and right index finger, opposed, press simultaneously the right and left sides of the nostrils (Fig. 20). This improves the effectiveness of the next process by limbering the dilator naris muscles (Fig. 21). Each pressure application should last three

seconds. Repeat three times.

Stretch the nostrils by dilating them and inhaling with them dilated for ten seconds (Fig. 22). Then, relaxing the nostrils, quietly exhale a little at a time for five seconds. Sudden exhalation greatly reduces the effectiveness of this exercise. Repeat three times. This treatment makes breathing smoother and improves stamina.

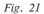
Fig. 20

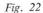
Fig. 21

Fig. 22

stretching the dilatator
naris muscle

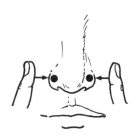

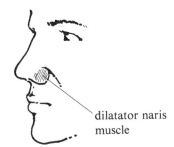
dilatator naris
muscle

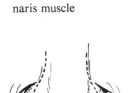

● *Stretching for the Eyes*
These stretching exercise, all performed with the index finger, on the nail of which is placed the digital ball of the middle finger, are repeated up-down movements. They are performed first on the points between the nose and the inner tips of the eyes, next on the points on the middle of the eyebrows in the supraorbital region and in the infraorbital region, and finally on the points in the temples on a level with the region between the outer tips of the eyes and the eyebrows (Fig. 23). Up-down motions should be performed simultaneously on the left and right sides for one second on each point and should be repeated three times (Fig. 24).

Next, rotate both eyeballs slowly first ten times to the left then ten times to the right (Figs. 25 and 26). Repeat ten times for each direction at a faster tempo. This stretching exercises invigorates the eyes and limbers the optical muscles.

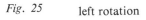
Fig. 23

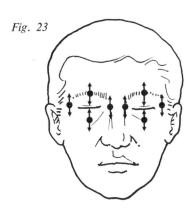

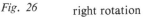
Fig. 24

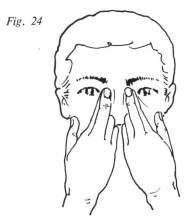

Fig. 25   left rotation

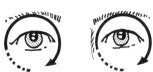

Fig. 26   right rotation

● *Stretching the Jaw*

Stretch the entire jaw by thrusting the lower lips forward (Fig. 27). Hold for ten seconds, relax for five seconds, and repeat three times.

● *Overall Facial Stretching*

Spread the fingers of the right hand slightly and, placing the center of the palm over the tip of the nose, cover as much of the face as possible with the hand. Next, with suction pressure, closing the fingers of the right hand slightly and drawing the facial skin upward with the digital balls and the bases of the fingers, contract the whole face—brows, eyes, nose, and mouth (Figs. 28 and 29). Hold this for ten seconds. Release. Next stretch the whole face by raising the brows, popping the eyes, flaring the nostrils, opening the mouth as wide as possible, and sticking out the tongue (Fig. 30). Hold for ten seconds. Alternating contracting and stretching, repeat each three times.

Effects

These exercises improve facial appearance; regulate powers of vision; prevent nasal blockage, empyema (sinusitis), facial paralysis, and pyorrhea alveolaris; strengthen the teeth; and bring relief from toothaches and eye fatigue.

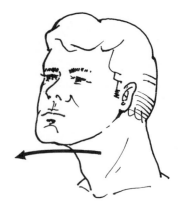

Fig. 27

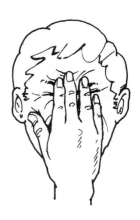

Fig. 28

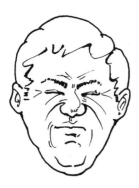

Fig. 29

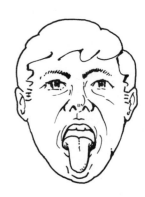

Fig. 30

8. Shiatsu and Stretching for the Chest

● *Shiatsu*

Muscles in the thoracic region include the external intercostal muscles, which are near the surface and raise the ribs during inhalation (Figs. 1 and 2), and the internal intercostal muscles, which are below the external intercostal muscles and lower the ribs during exhalation (Figs. 3 and 4).

Shiatsu pressure applied between ribs limbers these muscles. There are six rows of four

Fig. 1

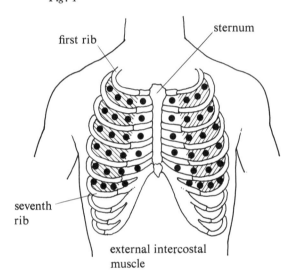

first rib
sternum
seventh rib
external intercostal muscle

Fig. 2

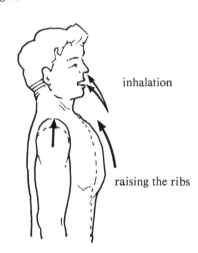

inhalation
raising the ribs

Fig. 3

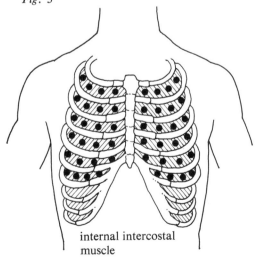

internal intercostal muscle

Fig. 4

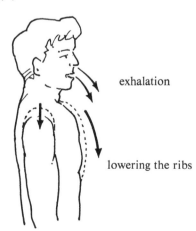

exhalation
lowering the ribs

Fig. 5

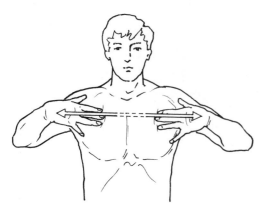

superior part of the intercostal muscle

Fig. 6

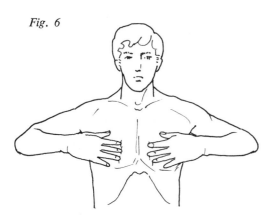

inferior part of the intercostal muscle

shiatsu-pressure points on each side of the chest. Treatment begins with the upper part of ribs one through four. With the index, middle, and fourth fingers of both hands spread slightly and placed at the right and left edges of the sternum, put the index fingers between the first and second ribs on each side, the middle fingers between the second and third ribs, and the fourth fingers between the third and fourth ribs. Simultaneously press with these fingers each of the four points on the right and left sides in the lines leading directly to the sides. Each application should last for three seconds. Perform the same treatment with the fingers placed between the fourth and fifth, fifth and sixth, and sixth and seventh ribs. Repeat three times.

● *Stretching*

Place the digital balls of the index, middle, and fourth fingers of each hand on the intercostal muscles between the first and second, the second and third, and the third and fourth ribs adjacent to the sternum. Simultaneously on both sides, slide the fingers toward the outside of the body, extending them as you go. When they have reached the external limits, inhaling,

Fig. 7

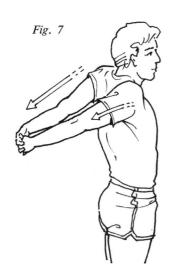

Fig. 8

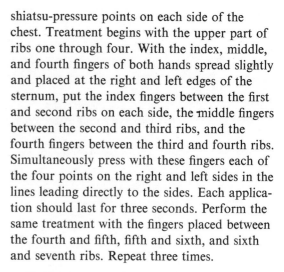

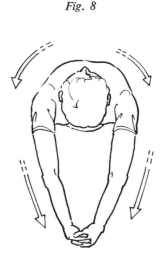

hold the stretched position for ten seconds (Fig. 5). For five more seconds, gently exhale. Repeat three times. Perform the same kind of stretching on the intercostal muscles between the fourth and fifth, fifth and sixth, and sixth and seventh ribs (Fig. 6). Then, inhaling deeply, hold your breath for ten seconds. Then relax by gently exhaling for five seconds (see Figs. 2 and 4). Repeat this inhaling-stretching three times.

To stretch the pectoralis major and intercostal muscles, extend your arms behind your back and interlock the fingers of both hands, palms inward. Stretch both arms downward and thus thrust your chest forward (Figs. 7 and 8). Hold the position ten seconds then release and relax. Repeat three times.

Next, with feet together, stand slightly in front of a door. Extending your arms rearward, grip one side of the door jamb in each hand. Lean as far as possible from this position without moving your feet (Fig. 9). Hold for fifteen seconds. Repeat three times.

These stretching exercises limber intercostal and pectoralis major muscles and make respiration smoother.

Effects

This therapy prevents intercostal neuralgia, bronchial asthma, and heartburn; stimulates the functioning of the heart; regulates respiration; and, in women, improves the appearance of the breasts.

Fig. 9

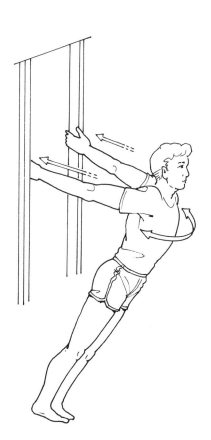

9.   Shiatsu and Stretching for the Abdominal Region

Fig. 1

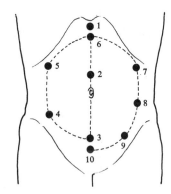

Fig. 2·

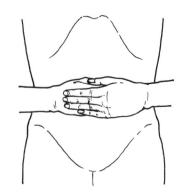

• *Shiatsu for the Abdomen* (*Digestive Organs and Abdominal Muscles*)

Fig. 3

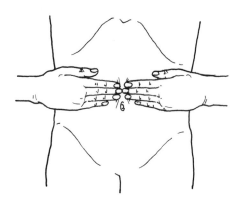

Improving digestion and absorption is of the greatest importance in transporting nutrients to the muscles, bones, and other organs of the body and thus in regulating the functioning of the internal organs. In this connection, shiatsu and stretching for the abdominal region are extremely effective. But neither should be performed when the stomach is completely empty nor immediately after a meal when it is full.

All of these treatments are performed lying on the back. The first treatment is pressure applied to the abdomen with both hands, left on top of right. The first point is directly below the diaphragm. The second is over the small intestine, the third over the urinary bladder, the fourth over the ascending colon, the fifth over the liver, the sixth over the transverse colon, the seventh over the pancreas, the eighth over the descending colon, the ninth over the sigmoid colon, and the tenth over the rectum. They are arranged first in a descending line straight down the center of the abdomen and then in a clockwise circle (Fig. 1). Press each point for three seconds and repeat three times (Fig. 2). In all shiatsu for the abdomen, pressure must be synchronized with breathing. Inhalation precedes pressure, and pressure is applied during exhalation.

When pressure application with overlapped hands has been completed, repeat applications on all of the same points with the tips of the index, middle, and fourth fingers of both hands (Fig. 3). Press each point for three seconds and repeat three times.

• *Shiatsu for the Region of the Small Intestine*

The eight points for this region are aligned around the navel starting with point one to the right of and below the navel (Fig. 4). Press each

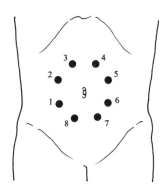

Fig. 4

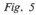

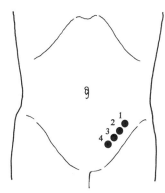

Fig. 5

with the index, middle, and fourth fingers of both hands—tips touching. Each pressure aplication lasts three seconds. Repeat three times.

● *Shiatsu for the Region of the Sigmoid Colon*
The four points for the region of the sigmoid colon are located on an inward slanting diagonal line to the left of and below the navel (Fig. 5). Press each for three seconds with the index, middle, and fourth fingers of both hands—tips touching. Repeat three times.

● *Shiatsu for the Rectus Abdominis Muscles*
During inhalation, the rectus abdominis and obliquus abdominis muscles, which perform the important role of protecting the internal organs, contract the abdomen. Limbering these muscles by means of shiatsu improves the functioning

of the internal organs and enables them to withstand stress better.

The rectus abdominis muscles extend vertically over the center of the abdominal region (Fig. 6). Pressure is applied for three seconds simultaneously with the index, middle, and fourth fingers of each hand to each of the two rows of six points on the right and left rectus abdominis muscles. Repeat three times.

● *Shiatsu for the Obliquus Abdominis Muscles (Externus and Internus)*
The obliquus abdominis externus muscles, near the surface of the body, lie on top of the obliquus abdominis internus muscles. Both sets run diagonally across the abdomen (Fig. 7). Six shiatsu points are arranged on lines that spread outward as they descend. Pressure is

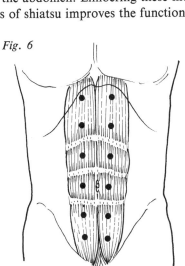

Fig. 6

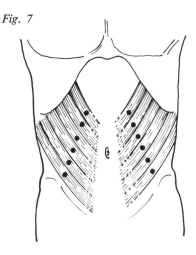

Fig. 7

applied with the index, middle, and fourth fingers of each hand simultaneously to each point in the two rows. Each pressure application lasts three seconds. Repeat three times.

● *Stretching for the Internal Abdominal Organs*
Stretching is performed for each organ in this region (see Figs. 1 and 4). First rippling palm pressure is applied in alternations of pulling and pushing on the region of the descending and ascending colons. The palm of the right hand is placed over the descending colon. The left hand is placed on top of the right. Then pressure is applied to pull the colon to the right side (Fig. 8). After this position has been held for five seconds, relax. Treat the region of the ascending colon in the same way (Fig. 9). Hold the stretched position for five seconds. Repeat,

Fig. 8

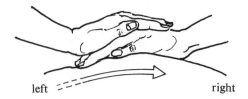

left   right

Fig. 9

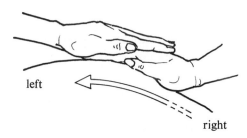

left

right

alternating on the descending and ascending colons, three times.

Circular stretching is performed on the small intestine. With the right palm pressed close against the navel and the left hand on top of the right one, execute clockwise circular pressure at a rate of one rotation per second (Fig. 10). Repeat ten times. It is important that the palm of the hand constantly remain in close contact with the skin of the abdomen.

Stretching for the stomach begins with ten seconds of vibration applied with both hands—right palm against the skin over the stomach and left hand on top of the right one (Fig. 11). Next, placing the tips of the index, middle, and fourth fingers of both hands over the center of the stomach at the height of the diaphragm, slide the fingers across the abdomen to the bottom of the lowest ribs (Figs. 12 and 13). Hold for ten seconds.

The stomachs of people suffering from gastroptosis will be located, not under the diaphragm, but below the navel. In such instances, the right palm is placed firmly against the skin over the stomach, below the navel. The

Fig. 10

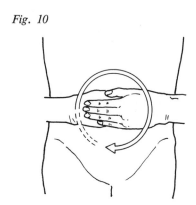

Fig. 11

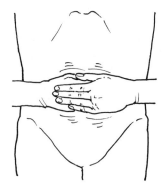

Fig. 12

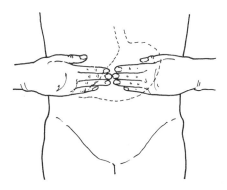

Fig. 13

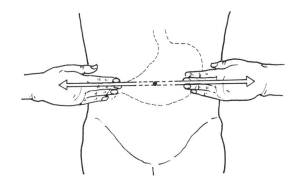

Fig. 14

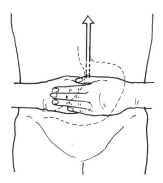

left hand is placed on top of the right one, and both are used to raise the stomach to the level of the diaphragm (Fig. 14). This stretched position is held for ten seconds. Repeat three times.

To treat the liver, place the tips of the index, middle, and fourth fingers of both hands at the center of the rib region on the right side. The palms of both hands are turned slightly inward and upward (Fig. 15). From this position, slide the palms of the hands right and left until the right hand is below the ribs on the right side and the left hand is in a slightly higher position on the inner edge of the left ribs (Fig. 16). Hold the stretched position ten seconds. Repeat three times.

Next, with the tips of the index, middle, and fourth fingers of both hands held close together

Fig. 15

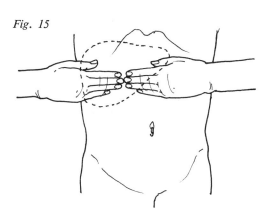

Fig. 16

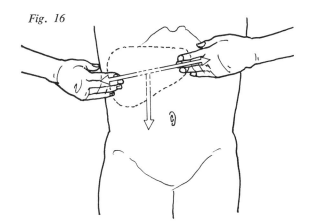

Fig. 17

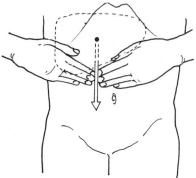

in the position shown in Fig. 15, slide the hands downward to a position close to the navel (Fig. 17). Hold the stretched position for ten seconds. Repeat three times.

To treat the urinary bladder, place the tips of the index, middle, and fourth fingers on the center of the lower abdomen, on a line with the navel and just above the groin (Fig. 18). With the palms of the hands close against the skin, slide the fingers straight to the sides (Fig. 19). Hold the stretched position ten seconds.

Finally, treat the sigmoid colon by placing the tips of the index, middle, and fourth fingers close together in the center of the region to the left of and below the navel (Fig. 20) and press the palms of the hands close against the skin. Next slide the fingers of the left hand diagonally upward to the side and the fingers of the right hand diagonally downward to the center of the body (Fig. 21). Hold the stretched position for

Fig. 18

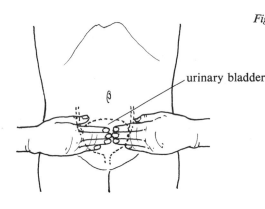

urinary bladder

Fig. 19

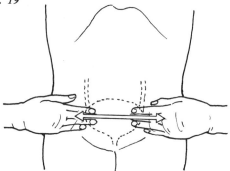

Fig. 20

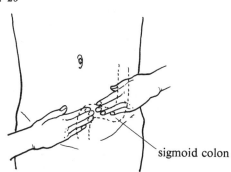

sigmoid colon

Fig. 21

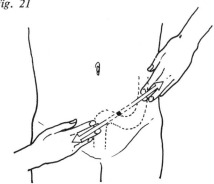

Fig. 22

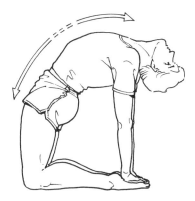

Fig. 23

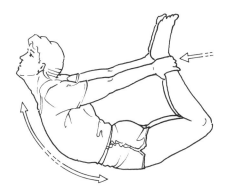

Fig. 24

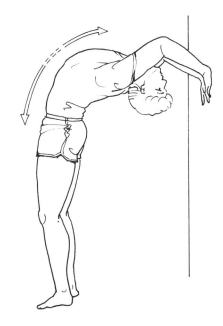

ten seconds. Release the hold you have with your hands and return to the starting position. Relax for five seconds. Repeat three times.

● *Stretching the Abdominal Muscles*
Kneel with both knees on the floor and the back held straight. Next lean backward and place the palm of each hand on the upturned sole of the corresponding foot (Fig. 22). Bending still further backward, hold the stretched position for ten seconds then relax for five seconds. Repeat three times.

Lying prone, raise your trunk and legs. Grip each ankle in the corresponding hand (Fig. 23). Bending still further, hold the stretched position for ten seconds. Release the hold you have with your hands and return your trunk to the starting position. Relax for five seconds. Repeat three times.

Finally, standing about fifty centimeters from a wall with your feet slightly apart, holding your lower body stable, bend backward till you face the wall. Put your hands, fingers turned downward, on the wall (Fig. 24). Bend your back still further and hold the stretched position for ten seconds. Remove your hands from the wall and return your trunk to the starting position. Relax for five seconds. Repeat three times.

Effects
This therapy regulates digestion and urination; prevents constipation, chilling, and gastroptosis; removes excess fat; brings relief from nervous stomach disorders; stimulates the functioning of the stomach, intestines, and liver; and improves the appetite.

Headache

Various things cause what is called the headache. Expansions of the blood vessels bring on vascular headaches, and contraction of the muscles causes catatonic headaches. In addition there are migraine headaches and headaches resulting from colds, hangovers, and hypertension.

■ *Treatment*

Shiatsu.　No matter what the nature of the headache, first begin with pressure applied to the part that is in pain. Pressure should be applied with the index, middle, and fourth fingers and should last for five or six seconds. Next apply pressure with the palm to the same place for ten seconds. Repeat three times.

When the pain has subsided somewhat, apply pressure simultaneously with the palms to the right and left temporal regions (Fig. 1). Each application should last for ten seconds. Repeat three times. Then apply pressure with both hands, one on the other, to the parietal

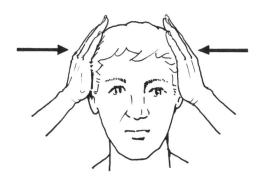

Fig. 1

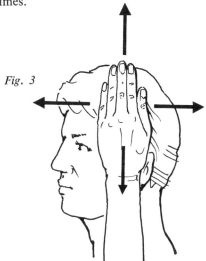

region for ten seconds (Fig. 2). Repeat three times.

Stretching.　Place the palms of the hands on the right and left temporal regions. Move them up then down alternately for five seconds each (Fig. 3). Repeat ten times. Leaving them in the same positions, move the palms forward then backward for five seconds each. Repeat ten times.

Fig. 2

Fig. 3

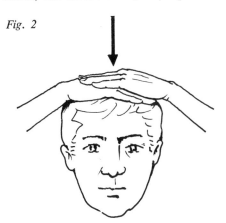

Finally, treat the parietal region. With the fingertips touching, place both hands on the slightly anterior part of the parietal region. Move the hands forward for five seconds (Fig. 4). Next, leaving them in the same relations to each other, move the hands closer to the occipital zone. Stretch them rearward for five seconds. Repeat the two stretchings alternately ten times.

Always cover the head with a clean towel or handkerchief before performing these shiatsu and stretching treatments.

Fig. 4

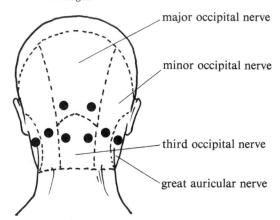

Occipital Neuralgia

In the occipital region, which runs from the nape of the neck to the parietal zone, are the following nerves: the major occipital nerve, the minor occipital nerve, the third occipital nerve, and the great auricular nerve (Fig. 5). On these nerves are points that cause pain when pressed. Pain on either one or both sides of the occipital region characterizes occipital neuralgia, which may be caused by tension in the muscles or ligaments of the occipital region, arteriosclerosis, hardening of fat, the whiplash syndrome, and so on.

Fig. 5   Distribution and Pressure Points for Occipital Neuralgia

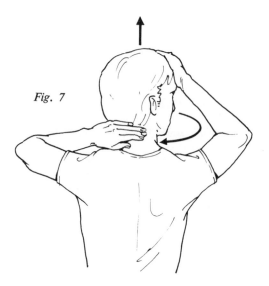

major occipital nerve

minor occipital nerve

third occipital nerve

great auricular nerve

■ *Treatment*
Shiatsu.   Shiatsu pressure should be applied in the vicinity of the point of pressure pain thoroughly and carefully until discomfort subsides (Fig. 6). It should be applied with the

Fig. 6

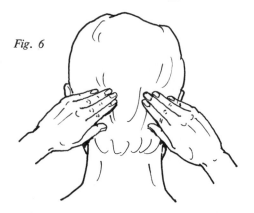

Fig. 7

index, middle, and fourth fingers. Each application should last for five or six seconds.
Stretching. When pain is in the left side, turn the face slightly to the right. Place the palm of the left hand in the nape of the neck, slightly to the left side, and the palm of the right hand on the right side of the forehead (Fig. 7). (The placement of the hands is the reverse for pain on the right side.) Stretch

Fig. 8   Distribution of the Trigeminal Nerve

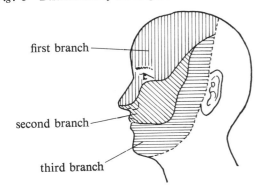

Trigeminal Neuralgia

As its name indicates, the trigeminal nerve, the thickest sensory nerve arising from the brain, has three branches (Fig. 8). The first branch is the ophthalmic nerve, the second the maxillary nerve, and the third the mandibular nerve. All three spread out over most of the face. Pain in any one is called trigeminal neuralgia. Points of pressure pain are located at the foramens where the nerves emerge from the skull. For the ophthalmic nerve, this is the supraorbital foramen; for the maxillary nerve, the infraorbital foramen; and for the mandibular nerve, the mental foramen. Causes of trigeminal neuralgia include vascular obstruction, nasal ailments, influenza, and dental inflammation.

■ Treatment
Shiatsu. Centering attention on the point of pain, apply pressure with the index, middle, and fourth fingers and vibrations as long as is required to bring relief. Pressure applications

upward with the hands and hold the stretched position for ten seconds. Repeat as often as is required to bring relief from the symptoms. The important point is not to take ten seconds to execute the upward move of the hands, but to move the hands upward and, exerting suitable pressure, hold the stretched position for ten seconds.

Fig. 9   Tender Points

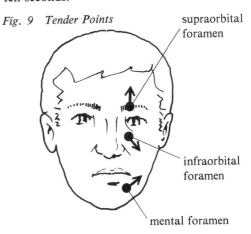

Fig. 10   Vibration

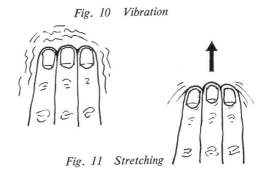

Fig. 11   Stretching

should last for five or six seconds (Figs. 9 and 10).
Stretching. With the index, middle, and fourth fingers, perform stretching on each point of pressure pain in the direction shown in Fig. 9. Each application should last for five or six seconds (Fig. 11). Repeat as often as needed. The important point is to keep the fingers pressed close against the skin and to press and raise and then, exerting a certain amount of pressure, to hold the stretched position for the specified duration.

Facial Paralysis

The facial nerve is a motor nerve controlling
the operation of the mimic muscles. Paralysis
in it causes symptoms to appear on one side of
the face. Though no pain is involved, this
paralysis results in facial distortion. For instance, if the paralysis affects the orbicularis
oris muscle, one corner of the mouth will
droop open, pulling the normal side in its
direction and causing the nasolabial sulcus
(furrow from the nose to the lip) to sag (Fig.
12). If the paralysis occurs in the orbicularis

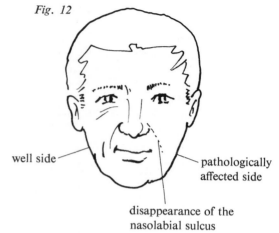

Fig. 12

well side

pathologically
affected side

disappearance of the
nasolabial sulcus

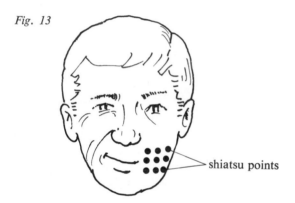

Fig. 13

shiatsu points

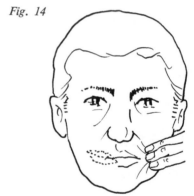

Fig. 14

oculi muscle, the affected eye will not close
completely (see Fig. 15). Paralysis of this kind
can result from external injury, influenza,
vascular obstructions, chills, excess exposure
to electric cooling devices, and so on.

■ *Treatment*
In the case of paralysis of the orbicularis oris

muscle, apply pressure with the index, middle,
and fourth fingers to each of the three rows of
three points leading from the corner of the
mouth along the zygomatic bone (Fig. 13).
Repeat as often as the symptoms require. Next,
with the index, middle, and fourth fingers,
apply suction pressure from the normal toward
the afflicted side of the mouth and hold this

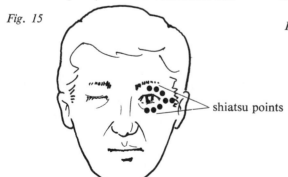

Fig. 15

shiatsu points

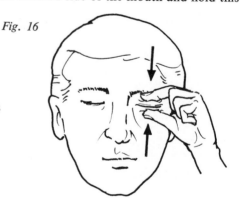

Fig. 16

position for ten seconds (Fig. 14). Repeat these steps as necessary.

In the case of paralysis of the orbicularis oculi muscle, with the index, middle, and fourth fingers, perform shiatsu on the two rows of three points in the supraorbital and infraorbital fossae and then on the two points at the outer end of the eye (Fig. 15). Repeat as necessary.

Then with the thumb on the lower lid and the index finger on the upper lid, close the affected, half-open eye (Fig. 16). Hold it closed for ten seconds and repeat as necessary.

Ringing in the Ears (Tinnitus) and Hardness of Hearing

Ringing in the ears can affect one or both sides. Causes may be numerous and often are unclear. Some major contributing factors, however, are stoppage of the external auditory canal with earwax (ceruminal impaction), hypertension, hypotension, arteriosclerosis, and the Ménière's syndrome. The shiatsu and stretching treatment outlined below effectively stops ringing in the ears and improves powers of hearing.

■ *Treatment*
To stop ringing in the ears immediately, insert the tip of the index finger into the auditory canal and move it back and forth to set up vibrations, which will reach deep into the canal (Fig. 17). Vibrate for ten seconds then remove the finger. This is done quickly. Repeat three times.

Next apply shiatsu pressure with the index, middle, and fourth fingers to the three shiatsu points on the temporal region behind and leading to the base of the ear (Fig. 18). These points are at the locations of the anterior auricular muscle, the superior auricular muscle, and the posterior auricular muscle.

Then grip the ear with the fingers and thumb wrapped around behind it. Press the carpal region of the hand firmly against the front side of the ear, which is completely enclosed with the hand (Fig. 19). Lightly but quickly twist the ear inward ten times and outward ten times. Finally with the hand in the same position, except that the carpal region is pressed still more firmly to close the ear entirely, vibrate for ten seconds. Quickly release the ear. Repeat three times.

Fig. 17

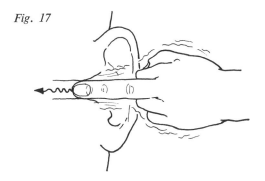

Fig. 18

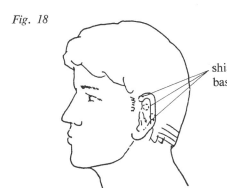

shiatsu points at the bases of the ears

Fig. 19

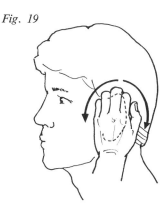

Nasal Blockage

Nasal blockage is caused by nasal fluid resulting from acute rhinitis, allergies, or sinusitis (empyema).

■ *Treatment*
Shiatsu. Shiatsu points for nasal blockage are the three points on the forehead median line between the brows and the hairline and the two rows of three points each on either side of the nose (Fig. 20). Apply pressure to the points on the forehead with the overlapped index, middle, and fourth fingers of both hands. Repeat three times. Pressure is applied to the points beside the nose with the index finger, on the fingernail of which is placed the digital ball of the middle finger. Applications, which are made simultaneously on the right and left sides, begin with the point at the inner end of the eye and continue to the ones beside the nostrils. They must neither be too strong nor last too long, for, if they are, they can aggravate inflammation of the mucous membrane. Press slowly and carefully for three seconds per application. Repeat from five to ten times.

Stretching. With the overlapped index and middle fingers placed beside the right and left nostrils, simultaneously pull downward from the corner of the eye and maintain pressure (Figs. 21 and 22). Hold this position for five seconds. Repeat three times.

Fig. 20

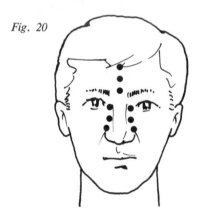

Fig. 21

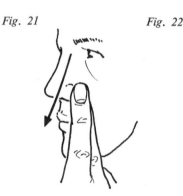

Fig. 22

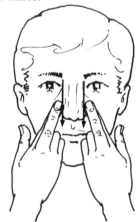

Insomnia

Most of the causes of insomnia are psychological, and the fear of being unable to sleep makes matters worse. Sleeping pills may be used on occasion but do not effect a basic cure and involve the danger of becoming addictive. For these reasons, insomnia presents serious therapeutic problems.

■ *Treatment*
Shiatsu. Most people who complain of insomnia experience stiffness in the general cervical (especially the anterior cervical) region, the suprascapular region, the interscapular region, the back in general, and the abdominal region (especially the diaphragm). Shiatsu treatment begins with the first point in the left anterior cervical region (Fig. 23). Pressure on this highly important point must under no circumstances be strong or last a long time. While being treated, the neck must be held natural, with its muscles relaxed. Each application of pressure, made with the thumb, should be slow and careful and should last three seconds. The first point in the right anterior cervical region must be treated in the same way. Once this point has been treated, restlessness, insecurity, and irritability should have vanished. It is effective to practice autosuggestion in treating psychologically determined conditions like insomnia. In this case, while carrying out shiatsu, you should instruct yourself repeatedly to sleep.

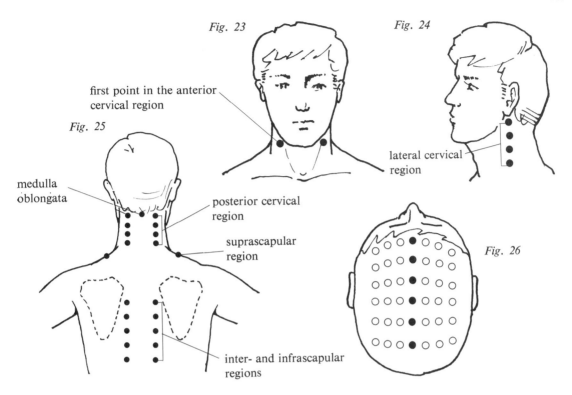

Fig. 23

Fig. 24

first point in the anterior
cervical region

Fig. 25

lateral cervical
region

medulla
oblongata

posterior cervical
region

suprascapular
region

Fig. 26

inter- and infrascapular
regions

Next, with the index, middle, and fourth fingers of both hands, simultaneously press the four lateral cervical points (Fig. 24). Each application of pressure should last three seconds. Repeat three times.

Press the point over the medulla oblongata with overlapped middle fingers (Fig. 25). Each application should last five seconds; repeat three times.

The last applications in the cervical region are on the two rows of four points in the posterior cervical zone. Press each point in the right and left rows simultaneously with the index, middle, and fourth fingers of each hand. Each application should last three seconds; repeat three times.

With the overlapped index, middle, and fourth fingers of both hands, starting with the median row beginning at the hair line, press each of the six points in that row (Fig. 26). Each application should last for three seconds. Repeat three times. After pressing the points on the median line, press those leading right and left from the sixth point, right and left

from the fifth, and so on until all six lateral rows of three points per side have been treated. Applications, which are made with the index, middle, and fourth fingers of each hand to the right and left sides simultaneously, last three seconds. Finally slowly press the sixth point on the median line with the overlapped index, middle, and fourth fingers of both hands. Each application should last eight seconds. Repeat three times.

Press the two suprascapular points and then the two rows of five points each leading from the interscapular to the infrascapular zones (Fig. 25). Begin with the left suprascapular point. Press it with the index, middle, and fourth fingers of the right hand. Each pressure application should last five seconds. Repeat three times. Press the right suprascapular zone with the index, middle, and fourth fingers of the left hand. Continue by simultaneously pressing the two rows of points in the interscapular and infrascapular zones with the thumbs. Press each of the ten points for three seconds and repeat three times.

110

Shiatsu for the abdominal region is performed lying face up. Beginning at the diaphragm, apply palmar pressure to the ten points around the abdomen (Fig. 27). Each application should last three seconds. Repeat three times. Next apply palmar pressure to the eight points around the navel (Fig. 28). Each application should last three seconds; repeat three times. Then, with overlapped hands

placed over the navel, vibrate for ten seconds. Repeat three times.

Stretching. Finally, lying prone with legs straight and arms above the head, stretch the upper body upward and the lower body downward as vigorously as possible (Fig. 29). Hold ten seconds. Repeat three times.

This shiatsu-stretching routine is effective if performed once before going to bed.

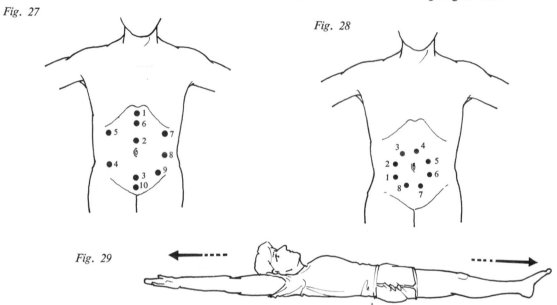

Fig. 27

Fig. 28

Fig. 29

Whiplash Syndrome

A difficult condition caused by modern vehicular traffic, the whiplash syndrome generally results from automobile collisions. The upper body of a person in an automobile involved in such a collision is suddenly thrown forward by the impact. Its own weight, however, throws the head rearward with the result that the neck is subjected first to hyperextension and then to hyperflexion (Fig. 30). When the impact of the collision is great, the head may be snapped back and forth violently several times like the tip of a whip. The resultant hyperextension and hyperflexion cause damage to the cervical vertebrae, ligaments, intervertebral discs, muscles, nerves, and blood vessels of the neck. Often in cases of whiplash

syndrome, no external injury is apparent; and X-rays reveal nothing out of the ordinary. Nonetheless, some degree of damage has been done to capillaries, vertebral ligaments, and muscles; and such symptoms as swelling and

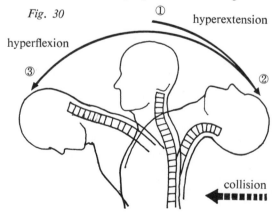

Fig. 30

inflammation will emerge in a few hours or on the following day.

Though it is important to wait until inflammation and swelling have subsided, to prevent

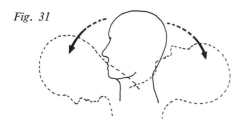

Fig. 31

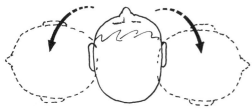

Fig. 32

Fig. 33

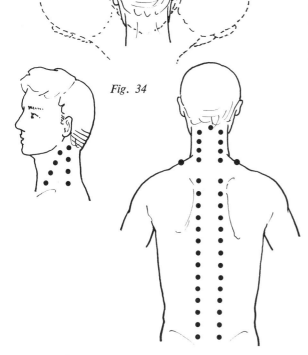

Fig. 34

persistent symptoms, shiatsu and stretching should be performed as soon as possible before twitching and contraction begin and the muscles stiffen.

■ *Treatment*

Shiatsu. First examine the condition of the muscles by moving the head backward and forward to extend and flex the cervical region (Fig. 31). At the same time, slowly rotate the neck to the right and left and bend it to the right and left to investigate the ease with which it moves (Figs. 32 and 33).

Next carefully touch the anterior cervical region, lateral cervical region, region of the medulla oblongata, posterior cervical region, suprascapular region, the zone from the interscapular to the infrascapular region, and the lumbar region and perform shiatsu on all points where the condition of the muscles requires it (Fig. 34).

Stretching. To perform stretching, sit in a chair or sofa with a low back and relax. Interlock the fingers of both hands and place the palms against the nape of the neck. Then stretch the neck by lowering the head rearward to an angle of thirty degrees (Fig. 35). Hold this position for ten seconds then return to the starting position. Repeat three times. Next lean the head forward to an angle of thirty degrees to flex the neck (Fig. 36). Hold this position ten seconds and repeat three times.

If stretching causes pain, stop and execute careful, thorough shiatsu on the region that hurts. Regularly and faithfully conducted, this

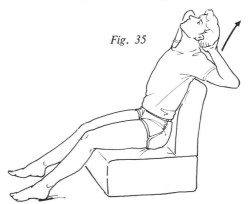

Fig. 35

combination of shiatsu and stretching can prevent lingering symptoms of whiplash syndrome and the psychological insecurity that accompanies them.

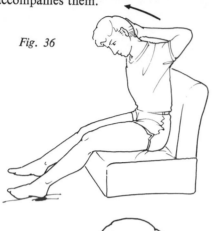

Fig. 36

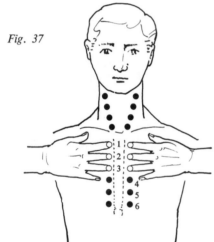

Fig. 37

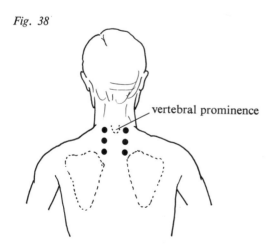

Fig. 38

vertebral prominence

Asthma

In asthmatic attacks, the smooth walls of the bronchial tubes contract (twitch) resulting in a respiratory difficulty called expiratory dyspnea. Occurring at night or in the early morning, attacks cause choking, distinctively wheezing breathing, and continuous coughing. Causes, which are various, include allergies; climatic conditions of temperature, barometric pressure, and humidity; psychological tension; and fatigue.

■ *Treatment*

Shiatsu. Begin with the left anterior cervical region (Fig. 37). With the left thumb apply shiatsu pressure to each of the four points for three seconds and repeat three times. Then treat the right anterior cervical region in the same way.

Two rows of three shiatsu points begin on the right and left sides of the vertebral prominence (seventh cervical vertebra), which can be felt when the head is bent forward (Fig. 38). The rows extend to a place immediately before the interscapular region. Reaching across your shoulders, with the index, middle, and fourth fingers of each hand press the right and left rows of points simultaneously (Fig. 39). Each application should last three seconds. Repeat three times.

In the chest, two rows of shiatsu points are located on the intercostal muscles on each side of the sternum (see Fig. 37). Beginning at the upper ones and descending, press the

Fig. 39

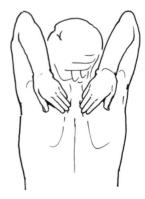

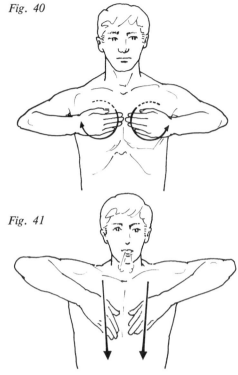

Fig. 40

Fig. 41

Finally, with the fingers turned downward and the palms placed against the chest, stroke the diaphragm downward vigorously and quickly as you exhale (Fig. 41).

Frozen Shoulder (Scapulohumeral Periarthritis)

A symptom of aging often emerging in people who are about fifty years old, this condition is actually a motor obstruction of the shoulder joints caused by lack of proper exercise. People who work at desks day in and day out and move their hands but not their shoulders are frequently victims. The posture their work demands obstructs circulation and deprives the shoulder joint of the lubricating synovial fluid it requires. The result is stiffness of the shoulder. When this happens, sudden unexpected raising of the arms or attempts to bring the hands behind the back cause sharp pain in the shoulders.

■ *Treatment*
Shiatsu. After performing thorough shiatsu to limber the area of the four points in the lateral cervical region, initiate treatment centered on the shoulder-joint zone (Fig. 42). Begin with careful shiatsu on the anterior, median, and posterior rows of three points each on the deltoid muscle, the four points from the suprascapular region to the shoulder

right and left points simultaneously with the index, middle, and fourth fingers of both hands. Each pressure application should last three seconds. Repeat three times.
Stretching. Place the palms of the hands closely against the chest in such a way that the tips of the index, middle, and fourth fingers of both hands touch on the sternum. Then execute outward circular palmar pressure ten times (Fig. 40).

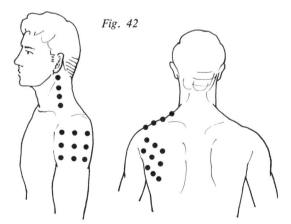

Fig. 42

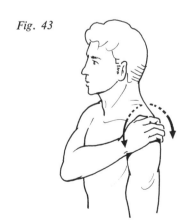

Fig. 43

joint, and the three diagonally descending rows of three points on the outer side of the scapula. Pressure should be applied with the index, middle, and fourth fingers.

Stretching.   Enclosing the shoulder with the palm of the hand on the opposite side, rotate the joint forward five times and then rearward five times (Fig. 43). Repeat this stretching exercise, alternatingly forward and rearward, three times. Next raise one arm, bend the elbow, and bring the hand behind the back. Place the opposite hand on the bent elbow and push downward (Fig. 44). Hold this position for ten seconds. Next stretch the arms diagonally upward. Grip the wrist of the arm being treated in the other hand (Fig. 45). Then, in three stages, raise the arm till it is straight over your head. Hold this position for ten seconds. Repeat three times. Do not bend the elbow of the arm being treated.

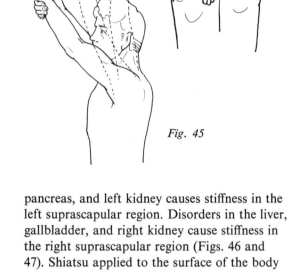

Fig. 44

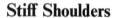

Fig. 45

Stiff Shoulders

The shiatsu and stretching, centering on the suprascapular region, outlined below is sufficiently effective for treatment of most instances of stiff shoulders, a condition usually resulting from fatigue. Some cases of stiff shoulders, however, are the consequence of pathogenic reflexes set up by organic disorders. For instance, irregularity in the heart, stomach,

pancreas, and left kidney causes stiffness in the left suprascapular region. Disorders in the liver, gallbladder, and right kidney cause stiffness in the right suprascapular region (Figs. 46 and 47). Shiatsu applied to the surface of the body to set up cutaneovisceral reflexes to correct these conditions will eliminate stiffness in the shoulders.

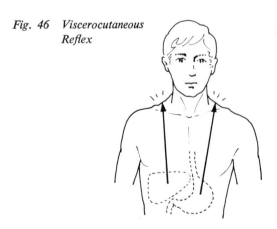

Fig. 46   *Viscerocutaneous Reflex*

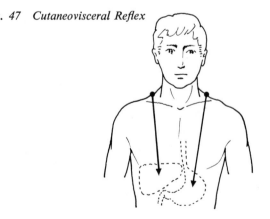

Fig. 47   *Cutaneovisceral Reflex*

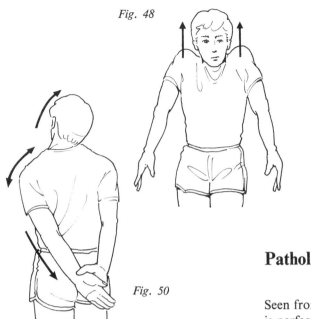

Fig. 48

Fig. 50

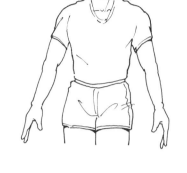

Fig. 49

■ *Treatment*

Shiatsu. First press the left suprascapular region for five seconds with the index, middle, and fourth fingers of the right hand and the right suprascapular region for five seconds with the index, middle, and fourth fingers of the left hand. Next limber the levator scapulae, supraspinatus, and trapezius muscles by applying shiatsu pressure to the lateral cervical, posterior cervical, and the area from the suprascapular region to the tip of the shoulder.
Stretching. First stand with both arms relaxed and hanging by your sides. Then lift both shoulders as high as you can (Fig. 48). After holding this position for ten seconds, suddenly relax the shoulders and let them return to the starting position (Fig. 49). Repeat three times. Then, bringing both hands behind your back, grip your left wrist in your right hand. While bending your head upward and to the right, pull your left hand downward with your right hand (Fig. 50). Hold this position for ten seconds and repeat three times. Then treat the right shoulder in the same way.

The treatment is even more effective if accompanied by shiatsu to both sides of the spinal column and to the abdomen.

Pathological Curvature of the Spine

Seen from the front, the normal spinal column is perfectly straight. In the lateral view, it consists of four physiological curves. The seven cervical vertebrae form a line curving slightly forward. The twelve thoracic vertebrae make a line curving rearward. The line of the lumbar vertebrae curves forward, and the sacral vertebrae and coccyx curve slightly rearward (Fig. 51). The entire column is a double S. When any of these curves is greater or smaller than normal, the result is one of the pathological conditions described below.

Lordosis. In this condition, the forward curvature of the lumbar vertebrae is abnormally great; and the pelvis thrusts forward (Fig. 52). Seen from the side, the normal forward incline of the pelvis is about thirty degrees. It grows larger if lumbar curvature increases and grows smaller if it decreases. In serious instances, the forward thrust of the pelvis imposes a burden on the lumbar vertebrae, thus causing lumbago. In addition, it can put pressure on the renal vein and thus cause albuminuria. It weakens the abdominal muscles, causes the internal organs to sag, and stimulates pain in the lumbar region.

Kyphosis (Humpback). This condition, which is sometimes called round shoulders, results from an exaggeration of the rearward curvature of the thoracic vertebrae (Fig. 53). Working with the back rounded for long periods keeps the muscles on either side of the thoracic vertebrae and of the back in general constantly extended and causes them to stiffen and lose their powers of contraction. The muscles in the front of the chest stiffen from being constantly contracted. And, if maintained for long periods, these conditions bring on kyphosis.

Flat Back. In this condition, the curvatures of the cervical, thoracic, and lumbar vertebrae are abnormally small; and, seen from the side, the spinal column appears to be almost straight (Fig. 54). This limits flexion of the upper body, causes stiffness in muscles and ligaments, aggravates the flatness of the back, destroys balance of the body's center of gravity, and brings about pain in the back and lumbar region.

Poor Posture. The rearward curvature of the thoracic vertebrae and the forward curvature of the lumbar vertebrae have combined (Fig. 55).

Scoliosis. Curvature of the spine to either the right or the left is called scoliosis. The curvature that occurs during the period of rapid growth at about the age of fifteen or sixteen is known as idiopathic scoliosis (Fig. 56). The condition is caused by torsion of the individual vertebrae. If the torsion is to the left, the spinal column will curve to the right (Figs. 57 and 58). As the malformation advances, rib protrusion of a kind never encountered in normal cases develops. Constant stiffness of muscles on one side of the spinal column can cause this kind of abnormal curvature. Excess load on one side only of the vertebral bodies of the individual vertebrae produces deformation that increases the tendency to scoliosis.

■ *Treatment*

Lordosis. Perform thorough, careful shiatsu on the Namikoshi points and on the points in the lower abdomen, the lumbar region, and the buttocks area (Figs. 60 and 61).

For stretching, first assume a comfortable

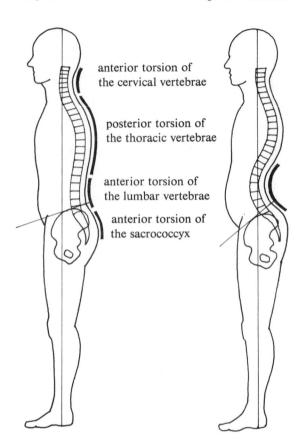

Fig. 51 Normal   *Fig. 52 Lordosis*

anterior torsion of the cervical vertebrae

posterior torsion of the thoracic vertebrae

anterior torsion of the lumbar vertebrae

anterior torsion of the sacrococcyx

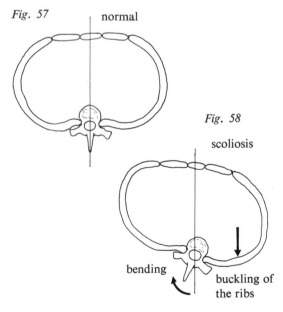

Fig. 57   normal

Fig. 58

scoliosis

bending

buckling of the ribs

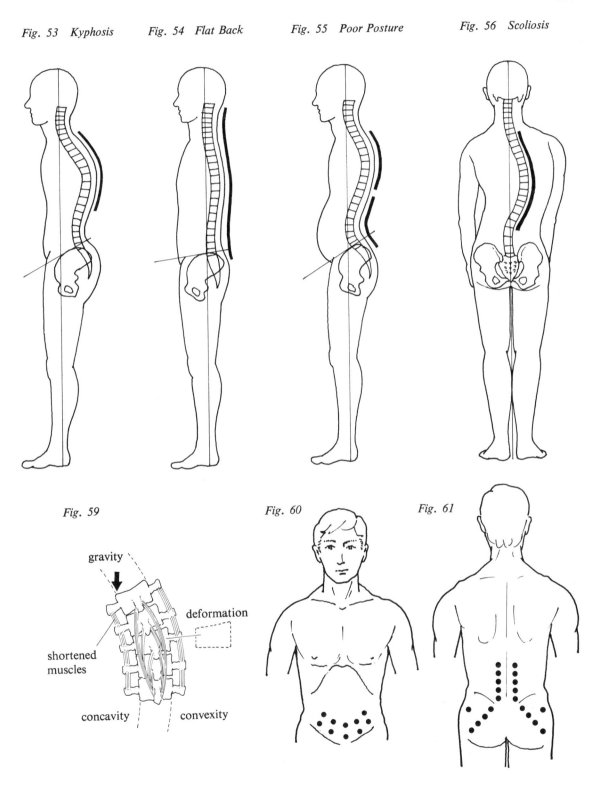

Fig. 53 Kyphosis

Fig. 54 Flat Back

Fig. 55 Poor Posture

Fig. 56 Scoliosis

Fig. 59

gravity

deformation

shortened
muscles

concavity

convexity

Fig. 60

Fig. 61

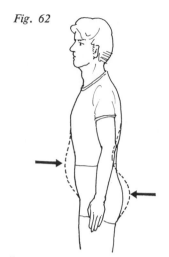

Fig. 62

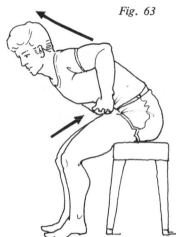

Fig. 63

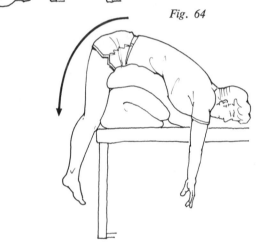

Fig. 64

standing position. Simultaneously contract the lower abdomen by pulling it in and contract the buttocks by thrusting them forward (Fig. 62). Hold this position for ten seconds. Repeat three times.

Then stretch diagonally upward by sitting in a chair, interlocking the fingers of both hands in front of you, and then placing them against the lower abdomen. While doing this, lean your upper body diagonally forward (Fig. 63). Hold this position for ten seconds then return to a comfortable seated position. Repeat three times. This exercise reduces forward curvature of the lumbar region by stretching the muscles of the back.

For the final stretching exercise, put two or three cushions, one on top of the other, on the forward edge of a table or desk. Lie across the cushions, with your abdomen on the highest part. This should raise your feet from the floor. Relax, with both legs hanging straight (Fig. 64). Stretch the lumbar region this way for twenty seconds. Return your feet to the floor. Repeat three times.

Kyphosis. First limber the muscles of the back with shiatsu in the region of the thoracic vertebrae from the interscapular to the infrascapular zone (Fig. 65). Then limber the muscles of the chest region, the diaphragm, and the abdominal region with thorough shiatsu on all their points (Fig. 66). Shiatsu on the back is especially important and should

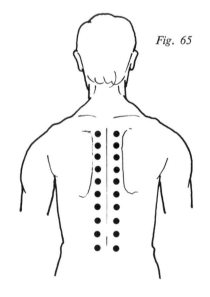

Fig. 65

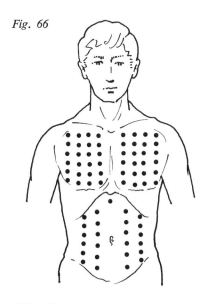

Fig. 66

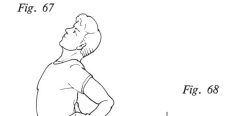

Fig. 67

Fig. 68

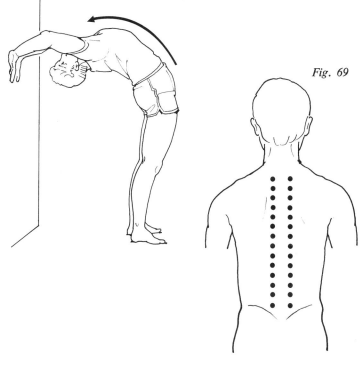

Fig. 69

be performed in standing, kneeling, or sitting positions daily. The following treatment will heighten the effectiveness of this treatment. Seated on a stool, bring your hands around your back and place both thumbs as high on the back as possible. Pressing simultaneously downward with both thumbs, bend your upper body rearward (Fig. 67).

For stretching, stand facing forward about forty centimeters from a wall. Bending backward, place both palms flat against the wall (Fig. 68). Hold this position for ten seconds then return to the starting position. Repeat three times. This strengthens the muscles of the back by stretching the anterior part of the trunk and contracting the back.

Flat Back. Points for shiatsu are concentrated on each side of the spinal column from the interscapular to the infrascapular and lumbar regions (Fig. 69). Direct the pressure toward the front of the body and bend the back by leaning the upper body slightly forward (Fig. 70). This exercise should be performed daily in either the standing, kneeling, or sitting position.

Fig. 70

Fig. 71

Fig. 72

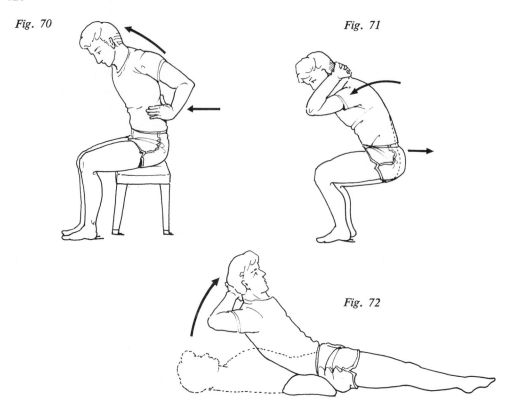

For stretching, standing straight, interlock the fingers of both hands and place them at the nape of the neck. Then, crouching by bending the knees, incline the upper body forward and pull the buttocks rearward (Fig. 71). Hold this position ten seconds. Returning to the starting position after each execution, repeat ten times. Next, placing a cushion or pillow under your lumbar region, lie face upward on the floor. Interlock the fingers of both hands and place the palms against the nape of your neck. Then raise your upper body (Fig. 72). Repeat ten times.

Fig. 73

strengthening the back muscles

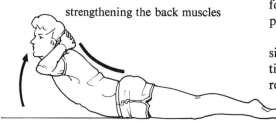

Poor Posture. After executing the shiatsu and stretching prescribed for lordosis and kyphosis, heighten the effect of the therapy with strong stretching of the back and abdominal muscles. First, strengthen the back with the following exercise. Lying prone on the floor with the fingers of both hands interlocked and the palms placed against the nape of the neck, raise the upper trunk (Fig. 73). Hold this position ten seconds then return to the starting position and relax. Repeat three times. Then strengthen the abdominal muscles by lying, face up, on the floor, placing the hands behind the nape of the neck in the same fashion, and raising the trunk (Fig. 74). Hold for ten seconds then return to the starting position. Repeat three times.

Scoliosis. Shiatsu is performed on both sides of the spinal column with special attention to the four points in the posterior cervical region and the ten points from the interscapular

Fig. 74

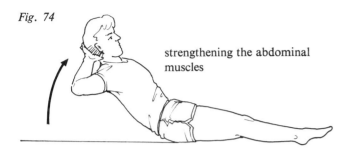

strengthening the abdominal
muscles

Fig. 75

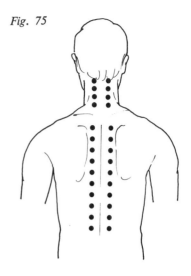

to the infrascapular zone (Fig. 75). Ascertain the degree of curvature by carefully locating the processes of each thoracic vertebra below the vertebral prominence (process of the seventh cervical vertebra) and placing a label of some kind on each (Fig. 76).

Stretching is performed in the following way. Sitting in a chair with the fingers of both hands interlocked and the palms placed against the nape of the neck, lean forward, rearward, and to right and left (Figs. 77–79). Then, gripping the back of the chair with both hands, rotate your torso to the right and left (Fig. 80). Each exercise should last ten seconds. Repeat each three times.

Idiopathic Scoliosis. This condition must be caught at about the age of twelve or thirteen. If it is allowed to continue until the age of fifteen or sixteen, it may advance too far to be correctable. Early treatment and preventative steps are the only ways to deal with it. Parents with children aged twelve or thirteen should keep a constant, watchful eye

Fig. 76

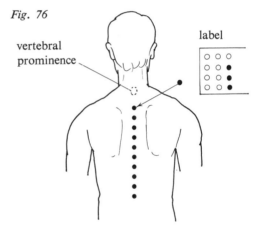

vertebral
prominence

label

Fig. 77 Flexion

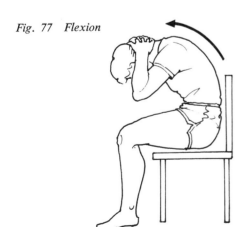

Fig. 78 Extension

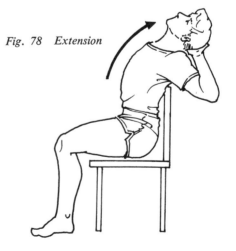

on the condition of their spinal column and perform shiatsu regularly on the muscles on the right and left of the spine to prevent imbalance. In addition, they should perform five or ten minutes daily of shiatsu on the posterior cervical and interscapular zones and have the children execute stretching exercises three times to extend the muscles of the back. The most effective prevention of idiopathic scoliosis is to teach this regimen to children and see that they carry it out themselves daily.

Lumbago

Ever since man began walking erect, the necessity of supporting a heavy head and torso has put considerable burden on the lumbar and scapular regions and has fated man to suffer from lumbago and stiff shoulders. Because of its numerous and various causes, lumbago remains a difficult condition to deal with. Some of its most typical origins are spinal irregularity, talipes varus (clubfoot), talipes valgus, contracture of the gastrocnemius muscle or the

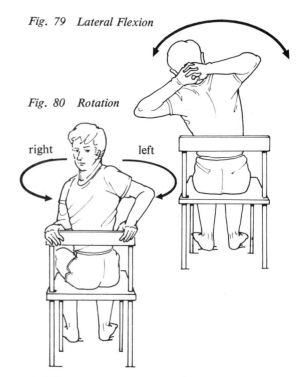

Fig. 79   Lateral Flexion

Fig. 80   Rotation

right   left

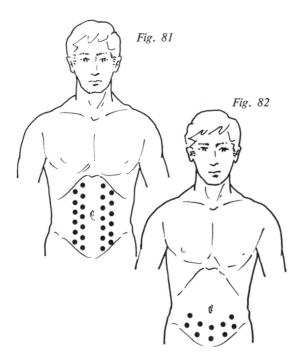

Fig. 81

Fig. 82

Achilles' tendon, and abnormalities of the sacroiliac joint.

■ Treatment

Shiatsu.   First, lying face up on the floor, perform shiatsu on the rectus abdominis muscles. The points are located in two rows on either side of the navel: seven points each in the inner rows and six points each in the outer ones (Fig. 81). With the fingers of both hands interlocked, apply pressure to each point, left and right simultaneously, with the carpal regions of both hands. Work from the top points downward. Treating the inner rows then the outer rows, repeat this shiatsu as many times as seems necessary. Then treat the same points with the index, middle, and fourth fingers of both hands, once again, pressing right and left sides simultaneously. For the abdomen, there are two shiatsu points on the median line directly below the navel and two more rows of two each on the right and left sides (Fig. 82). Working from the center of the body outward, press these points, right and left simultaneously, with the index, middle,

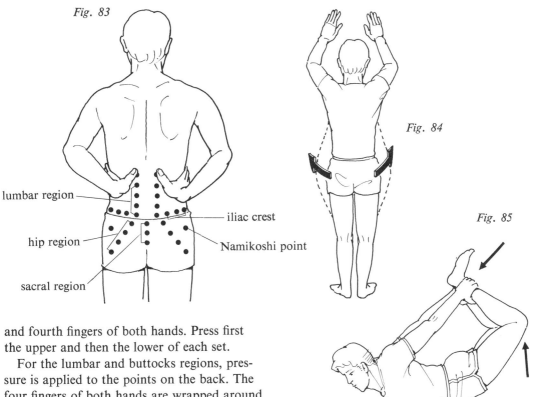

Fig. 83

lumbar region

hip region

sacral region

iliac crest

Namikoshi point

Fig. 84

Fig. 85

and fourth fingers of both hands. Press first the upper and then the lower of each set.

For the lumbar and buttocks regions, pressure is applied to the points on the back. The four fingers of both hands are wrapped around the body for support. There are two rows of five points each in the lumbar region, three on the iliac crest, the Namikoshi point, four points on the buttocks, and three on the sacral region (Fig. 83). With the thumbs, apply pressure to these points, right and left sides simultaneously, and in this way limber the entire lumbar and buttocks region.

Stretching. For stretching, stand forty centimeters from a wall, facing it and with both palms on its surface and with elbows bent. Further bend the elbows to place the forearms flat against that wall (Fig. 84). Next, without altering the positions of the arms, raise the left buttock diagonally to the left and then the right buttock diagonally to the right. This exercise stretches the pelvis. Hold each stretched position ten seconds. Repeat three times.

Next, lying prone on the floor with legs straight, grip each ankle with the corresponding hand (Fig. 85). Pulling the ankles, simultaneously raise legs and torso as high off the

floor as possible. Hold the raised position ten seconds. Repeat three times. Then sit on the floor with both legs outstretched in front of you. Stretching both arms forward for balance, lean your torso rearward and raise both legs off the floor (Fig. 86). Without bending your legs, hold both torso and legs at a thirty-degree angle with the floor. Balance yourself on your buttocks. Hold this position ten seconds before returning to the starting position. Repeat three times.

Fig. 86

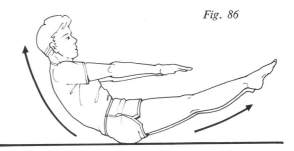

Standing with a wall about fifteen centimeters from your left side, with the fingers of both hands interlocked and the palms turned upward, raise both hands above your head (Fig. 87). Pulling arms and body straight up, bend your torso till your palms are flat against the wall. Hold this position ten seconds. Repeat three times. Then turning around execute the same stretching exercise to the right side.

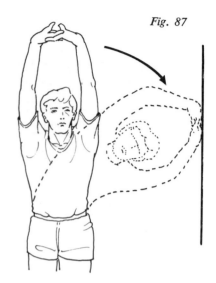

Fig. 87

Sciatica

The sciatic nerve, which arises in the lumbar region and extends throughout the lower limbs, is the longest and thickest peripheral nerve in the human body. Since it is close to the surface of the skin it is easily damaged. Sciatica, one of the most frequently encountered illnesses connected with this nerve, may be caused by chill, dampness, disorder in the lumbar vertebrae, or malpositioning of internal organs. Lasègue's sign is frequently used in diagnosing it. The patient lies face up on the floor with both legs straight and raises one leg. If pain results in the anterior side of the thigh when the leg is at an angle of forty-five degrees with the floor, the patient is suffering from sciatica (Fig. 88). Dorsiflexion of the leg will increase the pain.

Fig. 88   Lasègue's Sign

pain

pain

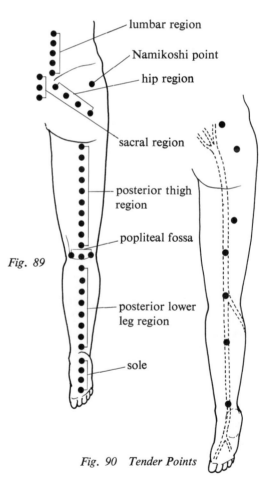

lumbar region

Namikoshi point

hip region

sacral region

posterior thigh region

popliteal fossa

posterior lower leg region

sole

Fig. 89

Fig. 90   Tender Points

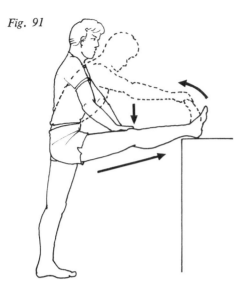

Fig. 91

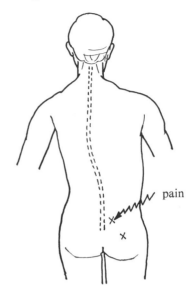

Fig. 92   Sciatic Scoliosis

pain

■ *Treatment*

Shiatsu.   First carry out thorough shiatsu on all the points in the lumbar and buttocks regions and throughout the legs from the posterior surface of the thighs to the soles to limber all the muscles passing in the vicinity of the sciatic nerve (Fig. 89). Since they develop easily in this instance, it is important to treat each of the pressure-pain points that arise all along the course of the nerve (Fig. 90).

Stretching.   For stretching, place the heel of one foot on a table or other object that is about hip height (Fig. 91). Press the thigh, immediately in front of the knee, with the palms of both hands, one on top of the other. Hold the stretched position ten seconds. Return to the starting position and relax. Repeat three times. Then dorsiflex the foot by gripping all of the toes with the hand on the same side and pulling them forward (Fig. 91). Hold the stretched position ten seconds. Repeat three times.

If sciatica becomes chronic, the body attempts unconsciously to avoid pain by shifting weight to the sound side, resulting in a condition known as sciatic scoliosis (Fig. 92). To prevent this, perform timely shiatsu and stretching to limber the legs and lumbar region and avoid chilling and dampness.

Cramps of the Gastrocnemius Muscle

Sometimes, without the person's being aware of it, fatigue accumulates in the gastrocnemius muscle—which accounts for the fullness of the calves—and the muscle stiffens. When this happens, exertion like that of running or swimming and sometimes movements no more violent than turning over in bed cause painful cramps in the gastrocnemius muscle (Fig. 93).

■ *Treatment*

Shiatsu.   In the case of cramps in the gastrocnemius muscle, sit quietly with the leg outstretched forward. Gripping the calf between the thumb and four fingers of one hand, grip the toes with the other hand and pull them forward to cause gradual dorsiflexion

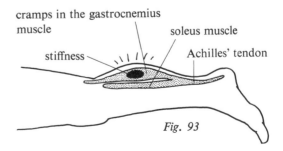

cramps in the gastrocnemius muscle

soleus muscle

stiffness

Achilles' tendon

Fig. 93

(Fig. 94). While doing this, applying pressure with the thumb and four fingers of the other hand, limber the calf muscle by quickly stretching it upward and downward and right and left (Fig. 95). This, combined with the following two stretching exercises, will strengthen both the gastrocnemius muscle and the Achilles' tendon.

Stretching. First, standing facing it, place both palms on a wall for support, advance one foot, and draw the other to the rear (Fig. 96). Move the torso forward by bending the knee of the advanced foot, while keeping the sole of the rearward foot on the floor. Hold this

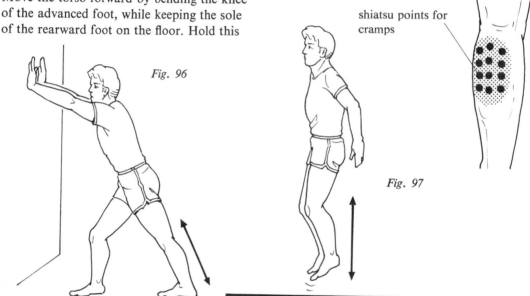

Fig. 94

dorsiflexion

Fig. 95

shiatsu points for cramps

Fig. 96

Fig. 97

position ten seconds. Return to the starting position and repeat with foot positions reversed. Alternating right and left feet in the advanced and withdrawn positions, repeat three times.

The second exercise is jumping on tiptoe twenty times, with the body completely relaxed (Fig. 97).

Constipation

The autonomic nerves regulate the functioning of the internal organs: the sympathetic nerves restrain and the parasympathetic nerves stimulate their action and work in mutual opposition to each other. When the balance of the autonomic nerves is upset, the parasympathetic nerves fail to function as they should. This dulls intestinal peristalsis with the result that assimilation becomes sluggish and constipation sets in. Irregular eating habits and habitual omission of breakfast can cause this condition, as can the side effects of medicines and psychological stress.

■ *Treatment*

Shiatsu. Lying face up on the floor, beginning at the diaphragm, first execute shiatsu on the points around the abdomen (see p. 96 Fig. 1). Follow this with shiatsu on the sigmoid

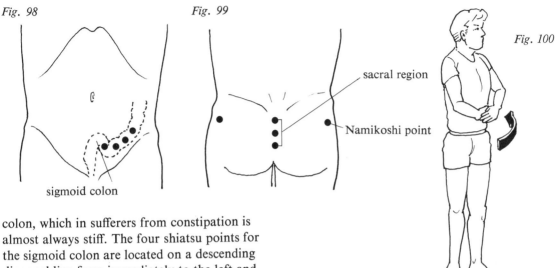

Fig. 98   Fig. 99

sigmoid colon

sacral region

Namikoshi point

Fig. 100

colon, which in sufferers from constipation is almost always stiff. The four shiatsu points for the sigmoid colon are located on a descending diagonal line from immediately to the left and below the navel to the region near the rectum (Fig. 98). Limber the colon by applying pressure to each point slowly with the thenar of the right hand. Place the palm of the left hand on top of the right while pressure is being applied.

Next treat the Namikoshi points on the buttocks and the three points in the sacral region (Fig. 99). With the thumbs and with the four fingers of the hand held to the side for support, apply strong pressure simultaneously to both the right and left Namikoshi points. Repeat several times. Next, with the index, middle, and fourth fingers of both hands, tips touching, starting at the first one, apply pressure to all three points in the sacral area. Repeat several times, always starting at the top and working downward. Then press each with overlapping index, middle, and fourth fingers of both hands until the pressure has penetrated well.

Stretching. For stretching, stand straight. Treatment is concentrated in the area of the sigmoid colon. First, with the palm of one hand on the sigmoid-colon area and the other hand on top of this hand, rotate the body to the left (Figs. 100 and 101). Hold the stretched position ten seconds. Repeat three times. Next rotate the body to the right in the same way. Hold the stretched position ten seconds and

Fig. 101

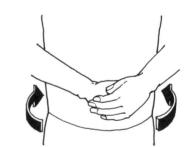

Fig. 102

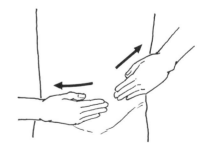

repeat three times. Then following the locations of the shiatsu points, with the hands draw the sigmoid colon simultaneously to the right and left (Fig. 102). Hold each stretched position ten seconds. Repeat three times.

Gastroptosis

To keep the stomach in its normal position, at the location of the diaphragm, above the navel, a certain degree of tension must be maintained in the abdominal muscles and walls. If this proves impossible, the stomach will gradually sink until it reaches the location of the pelvic canal. This condition is known as gastroptosis. Though in the early stage, no apparent symptoms manifest themselves, as the condition worsens, the patient will suffer from constipation, indigestion, and loss of appetite. This complaint is common in people who are constitutionally thin or have long trunks.

■ *Treatment*
Shiatsu.   Lying, face up, on the floor with the legs straight, execute thorough shiatsu with the palms and the index, middle, and fourth fingers on the whole abdominal region (see p. 96 Fig. 1). When tension has been eased in this area, continue to the lower abdomen immediately above the stomach and carefully execute shiatsu with the palms and the index, middle, and fourth fingers on the points in that

Fig. 103

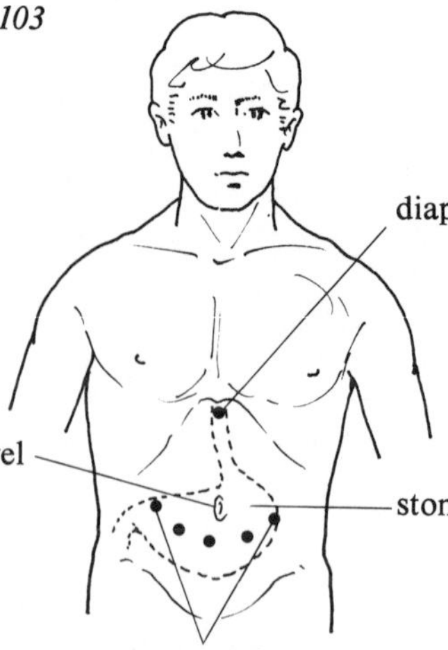

diaphragm

navel

stomach

shiatsu points

area (Fig. 103). Repeat several times.
Stretching.   With one hand on the back of the other, both horizontally aligned, and the palm of the lower one over the navel, execute penetrating vibration for ten seconds. Repeat three times. Then, moving in the clockwise direction, perform circular palmar pressure for ten seconds an application (Fig. 104). With one still on top of the other, place both hands over the position of the stomach, below the navel, and then draw them upward in a stretching motion (Fig. 105). Hold for ten seconds. Repeat this sucking pressure three times.

To strengthen the muscles of the abdomen, hooking the toes under the edge of a sofa or other convenient piece of furniture, interlock the fingers of both hands and put the palms

Fig. 104   *Fig. 105*

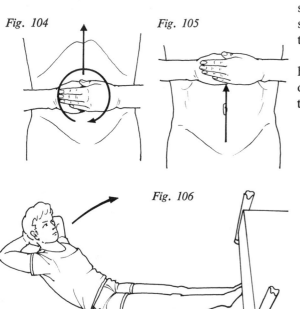

Fig. 106

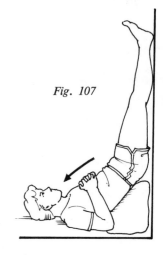

Fig. 107

behind the head. Then raise the torso and hold the raised position for ten seconds (Fig. 106). Return to the starting position and relax. Repeat three times.

Finally, rest your hips on a cushion placed at the bottom of a wall, lie face up, and place both legs, held straight, flat against the wall (Fig. 107). In this position, perform the sucking-pressure stretching described for Fig. 105 for thirty seconds. Repeat five times.

Gastralgia

Gastralgia, or stomachache, takes the form of dull pain in the diaphragm, nausea, heartburn, belching, and abnormal secretion of saliva. In advanced stages, the oral region breaks out in sores, the tongue turns white, and pain develops in the left shoulder and the back. At a still more aggravated stage, the patient suffers stomach cramps, or gastrospasms.

■ *Treatment*

Shiatsu. First limber the region from the diaphragm, which will be stiff, to the area immediately above the navel by performing palmar pressure on the three points there and repeating shiatsu with the index, middle, and fourth fingers (Fig. 108). Then press the right and left rows of three points each on descending diagonal lines in the infracostal region. The pressure should be applied with the index, middle, and fourth fingers of both hands simultaneously to the right and left rows. Repeat about five times.

The left infrascapular point and the three left interscapular points deserve emphasis and thorough shiatsu since they are places where reflexes connected with the stomach arise most readily (Fig. 109).

Stretching. Stretching is performed in the right and left infracostal region below the diaphragm with the index, middle, and fourth fingers of both hands but only after thorough limbering has been ensured by repeated shiatsu on the diaphragm and area above the navel. The index, middle, and fourth fingers of each hand are placed close against the skin beside the median line at the diaphragm and then are drawn simultaneously to the right and left toward the infracostal region (Fig. 110). The stretched position is held for ten seconds. Repeat three times.

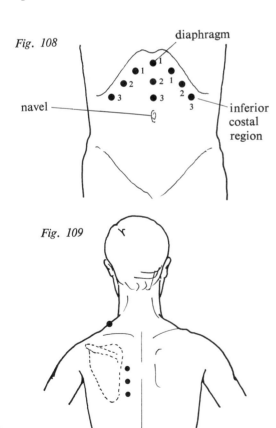

Fig. 108

diaphragm

navel

inferior costal region

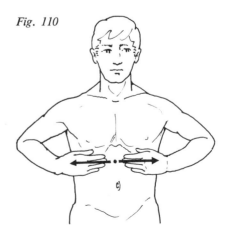

Fig. 109

Fig. 110

Strengthening the Heart

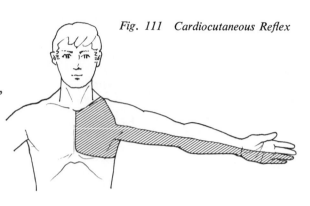

Fig. 111   *Cardiocutaneous Reflex*

Irregularity in the heart manifests itself mainly in the form of palpitations, shortness of breath, and an oppressive feeling in the left side of the chest. These symptoms are accompanied by dull aches and pains and numbness in the region from the left shoulder through the chest and the underside of the arm from the axillary region to the little finger (Fig. 111). This region, in which reflexes from the heart are revealed, is called the hyperesthetic zone. Shiatsu on it sends regulating reflexes back to the heart.

■ *Treatment*

Shiatsu.   Shiatsu is concentrated on the points in the hyperesthetic zone and begins with pressure applications, with the index, middle, and fourth fingers, on the suprascapular zone (Fig. 112). Each application lasts five seconds. Repeat from three to five times. This is followed by applications of pressure on the six rows of four points each in the intercostal regions of the chest. Each application lasts three seconds. Repeat three times.

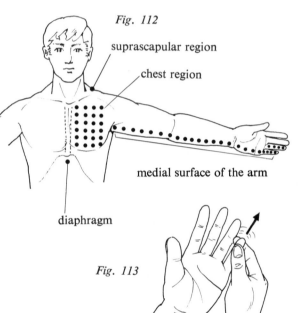

Fig. 112

suprascapular region

chest region

medial surface of the arm

diaphragm

Fig. 113

Next the index, middle, and fourth fingers of the right hand are placed in the left axillary region. The thumb is brought to the anterior side of the base of the upper arm (the position of the deltoid muscle) for support. Pressure is applied for five seconds and is directed toward the suprascapular zone. Repeat three times. Then press the tip of the right thumb against the left axillary region and wrap the four fingers of the right hand around the outer part of the upper arm for support. With the right thumb press each of the six points leading along the inner side of the upper arm to the cubital fossa. Each application lasts three seconds. Repeat three times. With the right thumb, turned directly upward and to the outside, press the point in the cubital fossa for three seconds. Repeat three times. Next are the right points in a row leading along the inner side of the forearm from the cubital fossa to the wrist. With the right thumb, its

tip directed toward the wrist and with the four fingers wrapped around the arm for support, press each of these points for three seconds. Repeat three times. Then press the four points in the hypothenar leading from the carpal region to the zone between the bases of the little and fourth fingers. Each application lasts three seconds. Repeat three times.

Gripping the little finger from the front and back with the thumb and index finger of the opposite hand, press each of the four points located on it three times. Repeat, gripping the little finger from the left and right sides.

Execute exactly the same therapy on the fourth finger.

Stretching. Stand with the left arm outstretched straight forward. Grip the tip of the left little finger between the thumb and index finger of the right hand. Pulling the left little finger forward, vibrate the whole left arm gently for ten seconds (Fig. 113). Repeat three times. Repeat exactly the same stretching exercise on the fourth finger.

Finally, perform shiatsu on the diaphragm with the tips of the index, middle, and fourth fingers of both hands brought together so that their tips touch. Each application lasts three seconds. Repeat three times.

Strengthening the Kidneys

Located on either side of the spinal column, in the region behind the navel, the kidneys function mainly in removing wastes from the blood and discharging them from the body in urine. When they fail to function properly, the metabolism is upset, the eyelids are swollen in the morning, and protein appears in the urine (albuminuria). If it advances, this condition can lead to nephrolithiasis (calculus in the urinary tract or vesical calculus).

■ *Treatment*

Shiatsu. The human kidney is about the size of the combined carpal regions, thenar, and hypothenar of the hand (Fig. 114). Interlocking the fingers of both hands behind the back and placing them on either side of the spinal column so that the left and right carpal regions are pressed against the body makes it possible to apply pressure from above to the positions of the left and right kidneys (Fig. 115). Apply sustained pressure for from five to eight seconds and, while doing so, lean the torso backward to add the weight of the upper body to the pressure and make it penetrate still deeper (Fig. 116). Repeat this palmar pressure on the kidneys five or six times.

Next, with both thumbs, pointed upward, and with the other four fingers of each hand wrapped around the sides of the body for support, press each of the three points on the kidney regions. Press right and left simultaneously, working from the uppermost point downward. Each application lasts three seconds. Repeat five times. Then, in short succession, press each of the ten points leading from the kidneys to just in front of the sacral region (Fig. 117). Each application lasts three

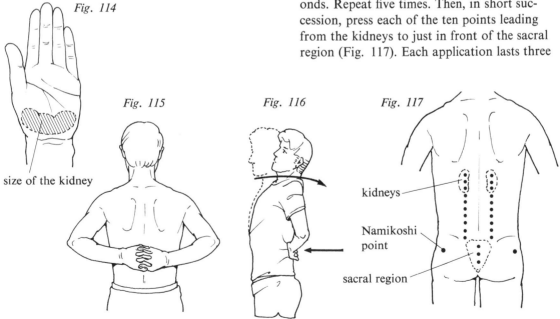

Fig. 114

size of the kidney

Fig. 115

Fig. 116

Fig. 117

kidneys

Namikoshi point

sacral region

Fig. 118

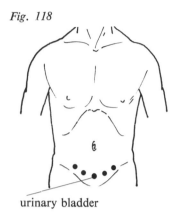

urinary bladder

Fig. 119

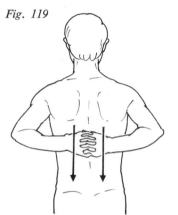

Fig. 120

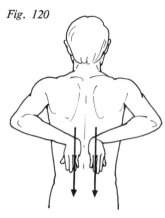

seconds. Repeat three times. Next, with the tips of both thumbs brought into contact, press each of the three points on the sacral region. Each application lasts three seconds. Repeat three times. Then, with the thumbs, simultaneously press the Namikoshi points. Each application lasts five seconds, and pressure should be strong. Repeat three times.

Next shiatsu is performed on the abdomen in the region of the urinary bladder. Lying face up on the floor with one hand on the other, press the bladder point, on the median line below the navel, with the palm of the lower hand (Fig. 118). Each application lasts five seconds. Repeat three times. Next, with the tips of the index, middle, and fourth fingers of both hands touching each other, press the urinary-bladder point. Then, with the index, middle, and fourth fingers of each hand, press the two sets of two points each on either side of the urinary-bladder point. Press right and left points simultaneously. Each application lasts three seconds. Repeat three times. Finally, with one hand on top of the other, vibrate the urinary-bladder point for ten seconds. Repeat three times.

Stretching. First, bring both hands, fingers interlocking, behind the back and press the carpal regions on the locations of the upper tips of the left and right kidneys. Then, with suction pressure stroke downward with both hands (Fig. 119). Without releasing pressure, hold the position for ten seconds. Repeat this stretching three times.

Finally, with the fingers of both hands pointed downward, rapidly stroke the right and left sides of the back simultaneously from the kidney to the sacral region (Fig. 120). Repeat three times.

Regular, conscientious performance of this routine will regulate the functioning of the kidneys and guard against hypertension, which is an immediate cause of kidney ailments. In addition to it, however, when the kidneys are weak, it is essential to get plenty of rest and to limit intake of liquids and salt.

Preventing Juvenile Myopia and Dental Caries

Myopia. Because they are called upon to read and write and perform other kinds of study and work to which they have been unaccustomed, first-year primary school children frequently develop pseudomyopia.

Fig. 121

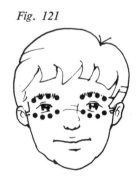

Fig. 122

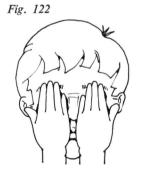

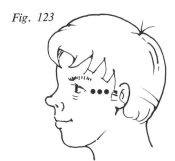

Fig. 123

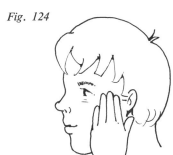

Fig. 124

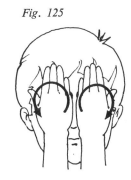

Fig. 125

Fig. 126

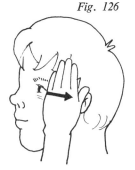

Fig. 127

Fig. 128

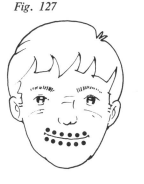

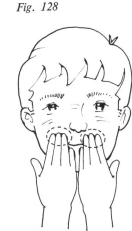

Rigidity in the muscles makes it temporarily difficult to control eye movement. To prevent this condition from developing, it is good to teach children the following shiatsu and stretching routine and see to it that they carry it out regularly every day.

Shiatsu is concentrated on the vicinity of the eyes (Fig. 121). First treat the four points in the infraorbital fossa. With the index, middle, and fourth fingers of each hand held together, press the right and left points simultaneously, beginning at the inner and working toward the outer corner of the eye. Each application lasts three seconds. Repeat three times. Next perform the same therapy on the four points in the supraorbital fossae (Figs. 121 and 122). With a pulling motion from the outer corner of the eye toward the ear, apply shiatsu pressure simultaneously to the three temporal points on either side of the head (Figs. 123 and 124). Each application lasts three seconds. Repeat three times.

Taking care not to apply pressure directly to the eyeballs, place the palm of each hand on the eye lightly and, simultaneously on the right and left sides, execute circular stretching (outward rotation) on both eyes (Fig. 125). Each rotation should last one second; repeat ten times. Next, putting the palms against them, pull the right and left temples simultaneously in the direction of the ears (Fig. 126). Hold the stretched position ten seconds. Repeat three times.

This entire regimen should be performed daily from one to three times.

Dental Caries and Pyorrhea. This preventative therapy begins with shiatsu on the anterior gums. Two rows of points on the upper gum begin directly below the nose and above the upper lip. Starting in the center and working outward to the corner of the mouth, press the right and left points simultaneously (Figs. 127 and 128). The fingers should lightly touch each gum position. Each application lasts three seconds. Repeat three times. Perform the same treatment on the points on the lower gum.

This is followed by short-interval stretching

on the upper and lower gums, beginning in the center and working outward. First stretch the upper three points, right and left simultaneously, upward for one second then downward for one second (Fig. 129). Repeat three times. Perform the same therapy on the points on the lower gum.

If performed regularly from one to three times daily, such preventative shiatsu and stretching are very effective.

Staying Youthful Longer

Wrinkled skin in the neck, especially the anterior cervical region, is an unfailing and unavoidable sign of aging. When the muscles in this region weaken, atrophy, and stiffen, transport of blood to the brain through the carotid artery fails to proceed smoothly. As a consequence, brain cells atrophy, functioning of

Fig. 129

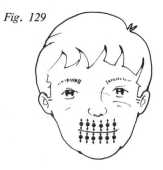

Fig. 130

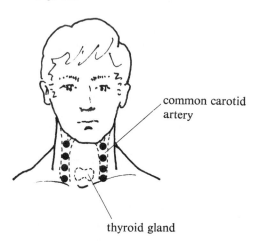

common carotid artery

thyroid gland

Fig. 131

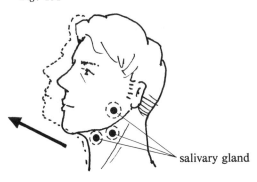

salivary gland

Fig. 132

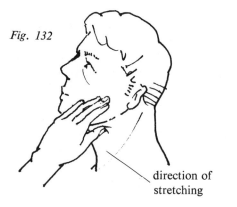

direction of stretching

the thyroid gland weakens, and daily actions become dull. In addition, the voice cracks, secretion of saliva becomes insufficient, and phlegm accumulates in the throat. In short, aging in the cervical region is directly related to aging of the brain and accelerates the debility of the entire body. Limbering the cervical region during youth is the secret to remaining youthful longer. Beginning in the cervical region, treatment extends to age-preventing points all over the body.

■ *Treatment*
First limber the muscles of the neck and stimulate the transport of blood through the carotid artery and the functioning of the thyroid gland by performing thorough shiatsu on the two rows of four points each in the anterior cervical region (Fig. 130). Begin with treatment on the left side and then treat the right side. With the index, middle, and fourth fingers of each hand,

simultaneously press left and right points for the salivary gland. The points are located below and slightly in front of the lobes of the ears (Fig. 131). Next, leaving these fingers in place for support, with the thumbs, simultaneously press the left and right points located slightly above the first anterior cervical point. There are two points on each side. Repeat three times. Leaving the hands in the same position, stretch the neck diagonally upward (Fig. 132). Hold the stretched position for ten seconds. Repeat three times.

Treating the medulla oblongata effectively maintains hormone balance throughout the body by influencing the operation of the pituitary gland (Fig. 133). Shiatsu is performed with the overlapped middle fingers. Each application lasts five seconds. Repeat three times. Then apply vibration to the same location. Only one application of ten seconds is needed.

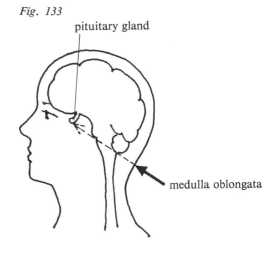

Fig. 133

pituitary gland

medulla oblongata

Fig. 135

medulla oblongata

pancreas

adrenal gland

kidneys

lumbar region

Namikoshi point

sacral region

Fig. 134

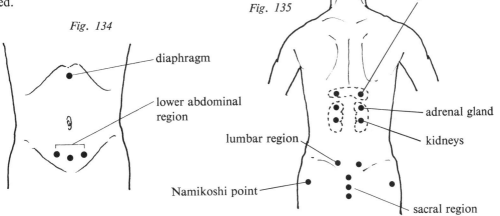

diaphragm

lower abdominal region

Treatment of the diaphragm and of the infrascapular region stimulates the functioning of the pancreas (Figs. 134 and 135) and thus, by improving secretion of insulin, helps control diabetes, one of the most prevalent of the so-called adult sicknesses. First, with the fingertips of the index, middle, and fourth fingers held so that they contact each other, slowly and carefully press the area of the diaphragm so that the pressure penetrates deep. Each application lasts five seconds; repeat five times. Then, pressing on right and left sides simultaneously with the thumbs, treat the supra-

scapular region. Each application lasts five seconds. Repeat five times.

Treatment of kidneys regulates their functioning; stimulates the removal of wastes, which contribute to aging; stimulates secretion of the suprarenal hormone; increases resistance; and relieves stress. For this therapy, interlock the fingers of both hands, place their carpal regions against the position of the kidneys, and apply pressure to right and left sides simultaneously. Each application lasts five

Fig. 136

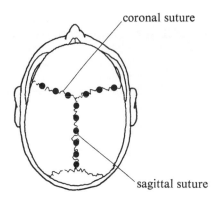

coronal suture

sagittal suture

Fig. 137

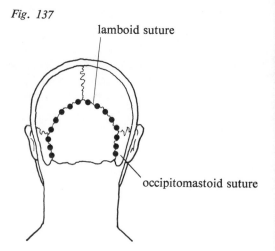

lamboid suture

occipitomastoid suture

Fig. 138

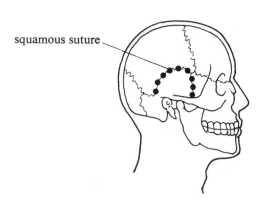

squamous suture

seconds. Repeat five times. Follow this with three ten-second applications of vibration.

Treatment for the gonads to stimulate secretion of the sex hormone involves pressure on the three points in the lower abdomen. With the fingertips of the index, middle, and fourth fingers of both hands held so that they touch, press the central point first. Then, with the index, middle, and fourth fingers of each hand, simultaneously press the two flanking points. Follow this up with palm pressure on the same position. One hand is on top of the other, and pressure is applied with the palms of both hands. Each application lasts five seconds. Repeat five times.

For the back, use the thumbs to press the points in the lumbar region, the three points in the sacral region, and the Namikoshi points (Fig. 135). In the lumbar region, each application lasts five seconds. Repeat three times. In the sacral region; each application lasts three seconds. Repeat three times. Each application on the Namikoshi points lasts five seconds. Repeat five times.

Finally activate the brain cells and prevent their atrophying by treating the head region, especially the sutures of the skull (Figs. 136–138). After thorough three-second applications of pressure on each of the suture points, carry out stretching as explained in Chapter Two (pp. 83–85) and follow this with vibration treatment (see p. 85).

● *Golf*

In these instances too, always precede stretching with thorough shiatsu on the part to be stretched.

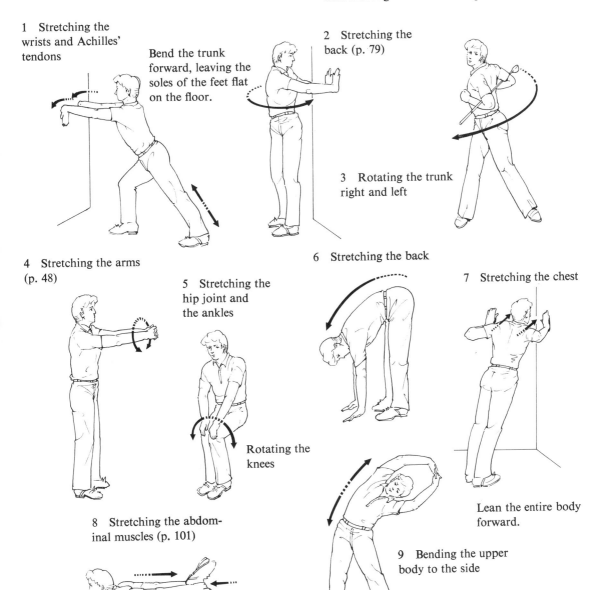

1 Stretching the wrists and Achilles' tendons

Bend the trunk forward, leaving the soles of the feet flat on the floor.

2 Stretching the back (p. 79)

3 Rotating the trunk right and left

4 Stretching the arms (p. 48)

5 Stretching the hip joint and the ankles

Rotating the knees

6 Stretching the back

7 Stretching the chest

Lean the entire body forward.

8 Stretching the abdominal muscles (p. 101)

9 Bending the upper body to the side

138

● *Baseball*

1   Stretching the
shoulders (p. 114)

2   Stretching the
arms (p. 48)

3   Stretching the shoulders
and elbows

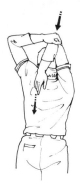

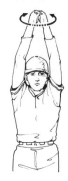

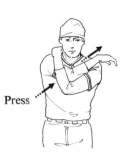

Press

4   Stretching the medial sides of the
thighs (p. 53)

5   Forward-and-rearward
stretching of the shoulders

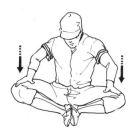

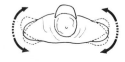

7   Rotating the
shoulders (p. 42)

6   Stretching the abdominal
muscles

Thrust both arms forward.

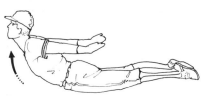

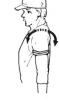

Bend the trunk upward.

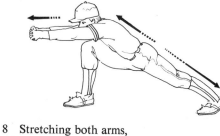

Keep both heels
on the floor.

10   Stretching the back
(p. 79)

8   Stretching both arms,
the back, and the posterior
sides of the legs

9   Stretching the
lumbar region and
the back

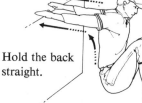

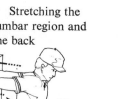

Hold the back
straight.

● *Swimming*

1 Stretching the back
(p. 79)

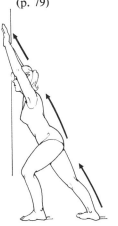

2 Stretching the back
(p. 79)

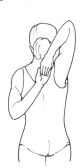

3 Stretching the back
(p. 79)

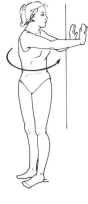

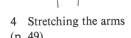

4 Stretching the arms
(p. 49)

5 Stretching the chest

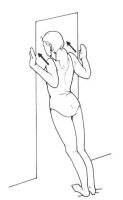

Lean the entire
body forward.

6 Stretching the abdominal
muscles (p. 78)

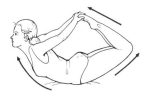

7 Contracting the back
(p. 119)

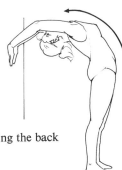

8 Stretching the anterior
regions of the thighs.

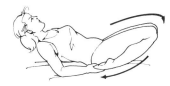

Pull the toes.

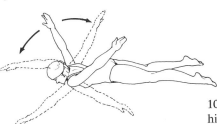

9 Rotating the shoulder
joint.

10 Stretching the knee and
hip joint

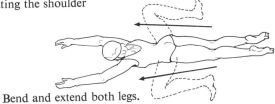

Bend and extend both legs.

● *Running and Cycling*

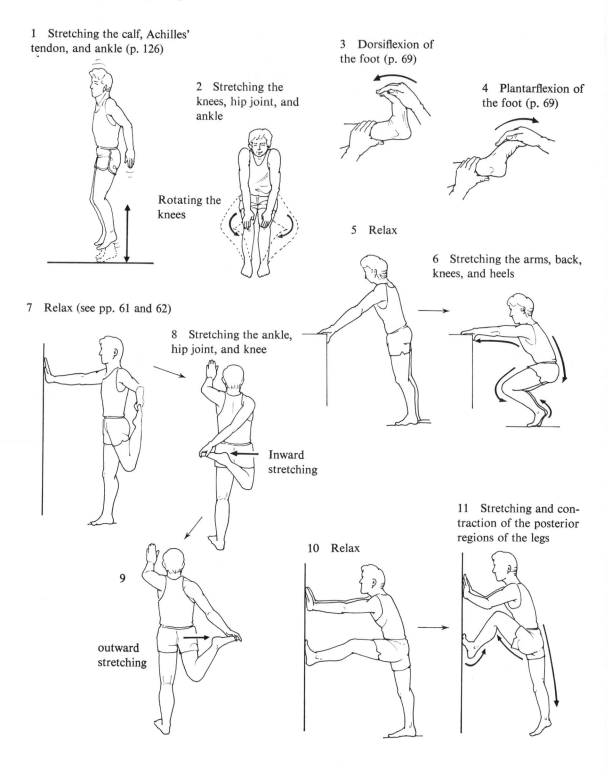

1   Stretching the calf, Achilles' tendon, and ankle (p. 126)

2   Stretching the knees, hip joint, and ankle

Rotating the knees

3   Dorsiflexion of the foot (p. 69)

4   Plantarflexion of the foot (p. 69)

5   Relax

6   Stretching the arms, back, knees, and heels

7   Relax (see pp. 61 and 62)

8   Stretching the ankle, hip joint, and knee

Inward stretching

9

outward stretching

10   Relax

11   Stretching and contraction of the posterior regions of the legs

● *Hiking*

1 Stretching the arms, back, shoulder, and back

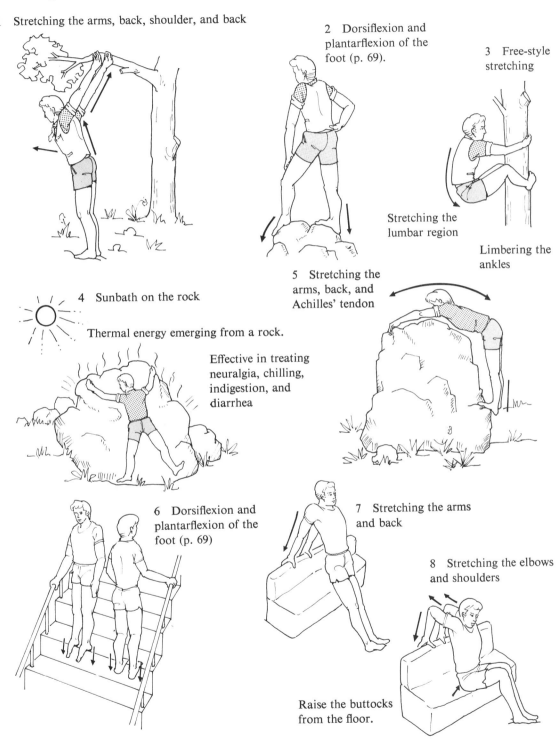

2 Dorsiflexion and plantarflexion of the foot (p. 69).

3 Free-style stretching

Stretching the lumbar region

Limbering the ankles

4 Sunbath on the rock

Thermal energy emerging from a rock.

Effective in treating neuralgia, chilling, indigestion, and diarrhea

5 Stretching the arms, back, and Achilles' tendon

6 Dorsiflexion and plantarflexion of the foot (p. 69)

7 Stretching the arms and back

8 Stretching the elbows and shoulders

Raise the buttocks from the floor.

Appendix B • For Better Appearance

1 Slenderizing the waist

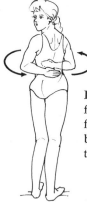

Pressing both hands firmly against the hips from the front and back, rotate the body to right and left.

2 Slenderizing the arms

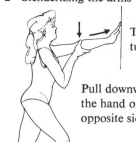

The fingertips are turned upward.

Pull downward with the hand on the opposite side.

3

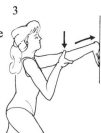

The fingertips are turned downward.

4 Slenderizing the posterior and medial sides of the thighs

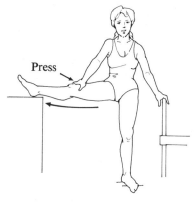

Press

5 Slenderizing the anterior and posterior regions of the thighs

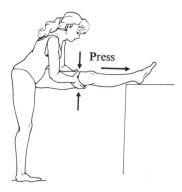

Press

6 Slenderizing the lower abdominal region

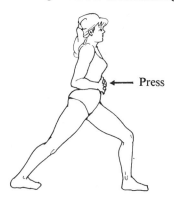

Press

7 Slenderizing the ankles and calves

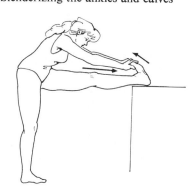

8 Improving the shape of the bust

10 Improving the shape of the hips

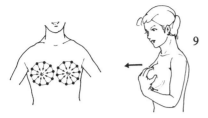

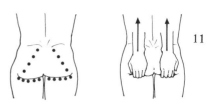

Appendix C • Shiatsu + Stretching in Daily Life

● *Before Rising in the Morning*

1 Both arms and both legs outstretched straight

2 The trunk raised

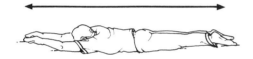

4 Both arms and both legs raised and rotated

3 Both legs held together and raised

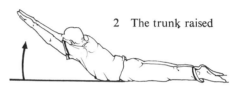

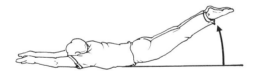

5 Dorsiflexion of the foot (p. 71)

6 Plantarflexion of the foot (p. 71)

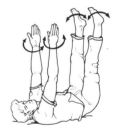

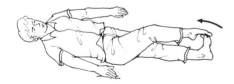

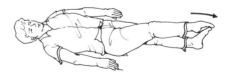

7 Stretching the medial side of the thigh

8 Stretching the back

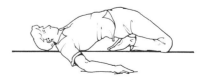

144

● *While Watching Television*

1 Shiatsu for the eye region (p. 89)

2 Shiatsu for the temples (p. 89)

3

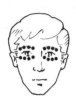

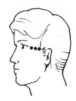

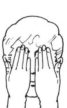

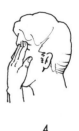

4

● *In the Living Room*

1 Strengthening the abdominal muscles (p. 128)

2 Stretching the lumbar region

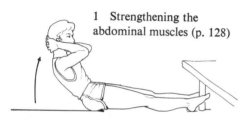

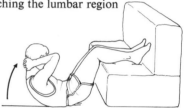

● *In the Office*

1 Stretching the shoulders

2 Stretching the back (p. 119)

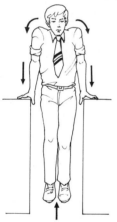

Raised from the floor

4 Stretching the back (p. 122)

3 Stretching the back (pp. 77 and 121)

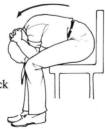

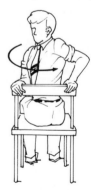

Index